Living with
Multiple Chemical Sensitivity

To my husband, Michael McCormick,
and to all who have learned to live
creatively and compassionately
with a loved one who has MCS

Living with Multiple Chemical Sensitivity

NARRATIVES OF COPING

by Gail McCormick

with a foreword by
PAMELA GIBSON

McFarland & Company, Inc., Publishers
Jefferson, North Carolina, and London

Disclaimer: The information in this book is not intended as medical, legal or psychological advice. Any theories, treatments, physicians, products or opinions mentioned do not represent endorsements or recommendations, and do not take the place of medical, psychological or legal advice tailored to specific individual conditions. Medical, legal and psychological advice should be obtained from licensed professionals in personal consultations. Products and or treatments that may be effective for some people may be harmful to others. Any persons using products or treatment modalities referred to in this publication, or who consult with or engage in treatment with any person or agency referred to in this publication, expressly waive any claims they, their heirs, successors or assigns may have now or in the future against the author or publisher arising out of any cause of action that may be created by the use of said product or service.

Part of the proceeds from this book will be used to provide MCS education, research and support to people who cannot pay for services.

Library of Congress Cataloguing-in-Publication Data

McCormick, Gail S., 1952–
    Living with multiple chemical sensitivity : narratives of coping / by Gail McCormick ; with a foreword by Pamela Gibson.
        p.   cm.
    Includes index.
    ISBN 0-7864-0887-1 (softcover : 50# alkaline paper) ∞
    1. Multiple chemical sensitivity.   I. Title.
    RB152.6.M345   2001
    616.07—dc21   00-46461
                                                                CIP

British Library cataloguing data are available

Front cover (clockwise from top): Carolyn Martin, Roy Bolbery, Tomasita Gallegos, Susan Molloy, John Pruitt, and Nicholas Weiss.

Manufactured in the United States of America

McFarland & Company, Inc., Publishers
  Box 611, Jefferson, North Carolina 28640
    www.mcfarlandpub.com

Acknowledgments

I am extremely grateful to the following people who made it possible for me to create this collection of stories: Michael McCormick for heart, soul, time and space. Laurie Riepe for clarity, compassion, and holding my vision. Nancy Ashley for belief in the power of story and helping to nurture the growth of this project in its infancy. Elizabeth Lyon for consultation and direction. Nicolette Rose for graphics with heart. My mother Phyllis Nelson for safe harbors, and for experiencing my world and the reality of MCS. Jim Nelson for Hallmark moments and transportation to Baton Rouge and Gulf Shores. Tammara Shaw for a chemical-free road trip to Dayton. Debbie Franz for a chemical-free Snowflake adventure. Michelle Franz for proofreading between a Russian song and dance. Ann McCampbell, M.D., for fine-tuning a medical overview and more. Lynn Lawson for resource comments. Cynthia Wilson and the Chemical Injury Information Network for contacts. Harriet Schatz and Shirley Ebert for open arms and wheels in San Francisco. Jennifer Kropack and Kathy Banas for editorial assistance and sharing my journey toward spiritual wholeness and environmental justice. All of the individuals who gave me the privilege of witnessing their stories, provided contacts and information, and nourished my spirit, including those whose stories are not published. All are a part of the collective voice creating a paradigm shift.

I am also grateful to: The growing circle of physicians, researchers, policymakers, activists and others who are responding to environmental health issues with right action. My family members and friends who honor my need for chemical- and fragrance-free encounters. And Bart Paff, Ph.D., for an incredible journey to joy and self.

Table of Contents

Foreword
by Pamela Gibson

How does one function in the face of the inability to tolerate the ubiquitous chemical exposures that are part and parcel of everyday life in industrial society? Most people understand traditional allergies that bring intolerances to pollens, dust, animals, and foods. Yet, the medical profession and the general public remain for the most part unaware of and unable to empathize with the inability to tolerate the products of industrialism that characterize Multiple Chemical Sensitivity (MCS). Pesticides, petrochemicals, fragrances, cleaning products, new carpet, and other substances laden with volatile organics are in use everywhere, and pose varying degrees of threat to those with MCS. Those with mild sensitivities may be able to survive well with moderate adjustments and avoidance of chemicals in the home. But what of those who have life-threatening reactions to common chemicals? One example is a woman who requires hospitalization and the use of blood thinners in order to recover from blood clots formed in response to particular exposures. Another is a woman whose heart stops if she encounters her most dangerous triggers. How does one risk access and the foraging of any kind of reasonable life under these pressures?

That many do, and that some of the most severely ill people have made valuable contributions through education, advocacy, and activism, is a testament to human resilience. Gail McCormick has captured in this volume the stories of those who live constructive lives in the face of the almost impossible. In my own work researching the life impacts of MCS I have found varying levels of financial, social, occupational, and personal disruption. MCS threatens one's livelihood, friendships, family, and personal happiness because of the limited access to places and people, and because of others' incredulous

1

attitudes toward the need for a chemical-free environment. Work and educational difficulties emerge because of the pervasive exposures to toxicants in the workplace and in schools. Most are aware that painters, factory workers, pesticide applicators, chemists, and farmers are exposed to poisons on a frequent basis. Yet schools, offices, stores, and other work settings regularly expose workers to pesticiding, renovations, toxic carpet, paint, solvents in cleaners and copy machines, and others' personal care products known to contain hundreds of harmful ingredients.

Over half of my adult research participants who reported becoming ill from a single chemical exposure encountered this exposure in the workplace. Unable to continue working, their loss of livelihood put many of them into a downward spiral that included loss of income, insurance, medical care, access to coworkers, and, as finances dwindled, even housing. The loss of work and the inability to tolerate toxins forces some into an invisible—sometimes totally housebound—role, marginalizing and silencing them. Culture continues on its chemical-dependent trajectory, effectively eliminating from view those who are harmed in the process. One labor leader has called this "cannibalistic titration."

The personal distress engendered by loss of access, work, relationships, and health can be overwhelmingly painful, and coping with MCS requires a level of personal resourcefulness that sometimes has to be acquired. Help from others can literally save some people's lives, as described by Susan Molloy in her narrative. Understanding from others and reasonable accommodations can sometimes spell the difference between making it and "going under." There is a tremendous gratitude on the part of those with MCS toward those who have taken the trouble to understand this difficult problem, and hope is generated whenever accommodations are offered. Professional conferences, city meetings, and even at least two university academic departments have become fragrance-free. Some family members value their loved ones over perfume and other chemicals, and thus allow for safe interactions with the MCS family member. My research participants cited the loving empathy of close family and friends as invaluable in helping them to retain their humanity in the face of this threatening disability.

Yet, unfortunately, few have the level of help needed, and people continue to suffer for lack of income, heath care, and safe housing. There is literally no toxin-free place to live in the United States.

Yet survival with MCS demands a clean environment, something that has vanished in a culture that is constructed by, protects, and benefits the dominant few. The dominant voices are the loudest, their experiences considered "the norm," and their needs and wants legitimized in a chemical-dependent capitalist/industrial culture. Those who deviate in any way be it through race, ethnicity, sexual orientation, lifestyle, socioeconomic status, or disability are marginalized to the extent that they are perceived as a threat to the economic and social status quo. In that it directly links an industrial lifestyle with illness, MCS may represent the greatest threat of all. For that reason it is not surprising that those with MCS face marginalization, isolation, and silencing as their health degenerates and they require cleaner environments in order to survive.

This book is extremely important in my view because it gives a forum to the voices and tells the stories of a "new" invisible minority who are casualties of our chemical-dependent economic base. Dr. Michael Lax, a specialist in occupational medicine, rightly insists that MCS is a product of industrial capitalism and cannot be understood independently of it.

A culture that cares for all of its people must hear the stories of all, as did Native American communities before the U.S. government pressured them into adoption of the European model of allowing a dominant few to do the speaking and decision-making for all. Today we are farther than ever from an all-inclusive model of community. In a country racked by racism, sexism, homophobia, and economic injustice, the stories of non-dominant people represent a crucial undercurrent or subtext necessary for a viable, holistic understanding of life experience.

Coping with a hidden, non-legitimized disability is one of the hardest things one can do in Western culture. Even so, people find strength, inspiration, and a sense of purpose in doing so. The people in this book have faced the void and survived, after which life is never the same. They do the impossible on a daily basis, and deserve the opportunity given in this book to tell their stories. In all of the world's myths the hero begins the journey with a loss or a calamity, which then propels him or her into an ordeal of moving, searching, confronting, fighting, making allies, and finally discovering the treasure that is needed for a re-integration of one's life. The people in this book are on that path. Forced out of consumerism, selfish purpose, and the sleep of the unaware, they struggle with daily lives that are poignant and beyond our cherished illusions. If one reads their stories and really listens, some new truths about our industrial lifestyle emerge. Time is short.

There is a strong motivation in the MCS community even under the most arduous of personal circumstances, to alleviate current and future suffering for others. Hence Susan Molloy describes doing disability advocacy work from her bed. Lynn Lawson has given us her book *Staying Well in a Toxic World*, a guide to safe living so well received that it has been heralded as the "*Silent Spring* of the 1990s." Dr. Ann McCampbell is a well-known disability advocate who has made consistent and admirable educational and legislative contributions. Irene Wilkenfeld works tirelessly for safer schools for our children. Terri Hansen's investigative reporting regarding Native American health and environment speaks to the importance of understanding the continued assaults on Native peoples. One does not have to be famous for one's contribution to be important. Meeting the challenge for survival and growth with MCS is cause for celebration. Going beyond this to help others understand the dilemma is often an important component of coping with MCS, and the best help for those afflicted comes from others who have walked the same path.

In desperation for health in a culture that offers marginal health care for many, and almost no health care for those harmed by toxics, those with MCS pursue many pathways for healing. What helps one often does not help another, and no treatment other than chemical avoidance has been shown to help more than a small subset of persons. Some have pursued spiritually oriented healing. In my view, confronting MCS on a psychological or spiritual level does not implicate psychological or spiritual variables as causal. Albert Einstein said, "The significant problems of the world cannot be solved at the same level of consciousness at which they were created." Therefore one does not have to believe that those with MCS have "broken hearts," psychological illness, "ecofear," or any other nonphysical origins for their illness to accept that some may be helped by "higher level" interventions. People integrate visualization, prayer, and other mind-body elements into cancer treatment. Yet cancer is clearly engendered by environmental toxins. The psychological research attempting to identify a "cancer personality" has been unfruitful, as have been efforts to identify a personality profile for those who develop sick building syndrome. Likewise there is no evidence that MCS is psychologically caused, while there are hundreds of toxicology studies that implicate environmental toxins in a myriad of negative health conditions such as asthma, cancer, reproductive problems, children's learning disabilities, Parkinson's Disease, psychiatric conditions, and others. The narratives of those with MCS are additional data for those who would listen—stories from those on the most sensitive end of the continuum that presage what may happen to more of us if we do not improve the way we relate to our earth.

It is my hope that this book will be used by a variety of people in some of the following ways, all with the aim of improving quality of life for those with MCS, and preventing others from developing MCS and other chemical injuries.

Others with MCS can read and relate to the journey of fellow sufferers, and derive hope from their survival, their coping, even their flourishing.

Policymakers can read stories of real people who face this risk of marginalization due to the brutal effects of everyday toxicant exposures, and take the experience of these people into their policymaking. Famous Love Canal environmentalist Lois Gibbs says: "Pollution begins in the boardroom."

People without MCS can become aware of the segment of the population that has become hidden from them because of industrial culture's refusal to moderate its rush to economic growth through exploitation of the environment. Rather than being a negligible small number, a rural household study showed that one third of the population reports some illness from chemical exposures, and four percent of people report becoming ill every single day from chemicals. This amounts to over 11 million people in the U.S. alone who suffer daily from chemically induced symptoms. Two other studies document MCS as a worldwide problem.

Health providers, including skeptics, can hear the voices of this hidden group and understand the tremendous efforts being made to survive, remain in contact, and contribute in spite of overwhelming odds. Far from using MCS as "secondary gain," the people in McCormick's stories have coped with losses that threaten to disintegrate one's lifestyle and identity, and managed to still come out on the other side with strength and compassion. Elizabeth Schuster says: "Life is love." Nicholas Weiss says: "If people who read my story have a child or niece with allergies, maybe they'll understand more and not just say it's nothing." And Herb Whitish: "I have an overwhelming need to help. That makes it more difficult for me to allow this to beat me.... My parents taught me to keep plugging away until the day I die, otherwise I don't live up to my potential."

Only by listening to those with MCS will we understand and empathize with their struggle. Out of this understanding needs to come the renewed values of respect for the natural environment and commitment to nontoxic living.

Pamela Gibson, Ph.D.
James Madison University
Summer 2000

Introduction

*Stories are protectors. Like our immune systems, they defend us
... against attacks of debilitating alienation... they prepare us for
the future and guide us in the present.. storying is a kind of root
medicine, a way for us to enter our depths and derive nourishment
from the fruitful darkness.—The Fruitful Darkness, Reconnecting
with the Body of the Earth, by Joan Halifax*

Your entire life is affected when one whiff of perfume, fabric
softener or fresh paint can result in a throbbing headache, brain
dysfunction, an asthma attack, a convulsion or a myriad of other
symptoms. Work performance, relationships and community ties collapse when your olfactory system is so heightened that you become
ill from the smell of laundry products on the clothes of someone
sitting all the way across the room. Fear overcomes you when suddenly carpeting, photocopies, car exhaust and other products produce the same effects, and the only way to protect yourself is through
isolation.

This is the experience of people with multiple chemical sensitivities (MCS), also known as environmental illness. People with
MCS are made ill by exposures to a variety of chemicals commonly
encountered in everyday life. Although the severe losses, profound
lifestyle changes and isolation associated with this illness can be devastating, little help is available for coping with the emotional and
social impact. Most of the literature on MCS focuses primarily on
the physical, medical, environmental and legal aspects. As a mental health counselor, a biographer and woman living with MCS, my
interest in addressing this deficit is both personal and professional.

This book is intended to give voice to the experiences of people
from all walks of life who live with chemical sensitivities. Their narratives describe many of the social and emotional challenges faced

by this population, illustrate some courageous and creative coping
strategies, and offer alternatives to isolation and hopelessness. One
story describes and validates the challenges faced by a healthy family member in relationship to someone who has MCS.

A Quest

All who live with MCS struggle with these questions: How do
you create a positive life when you no longer can socialize, work,
attend church or community events, shop, travel or sit in a movie
theater without unpleasant, if not serious, consequences to your
health? How do others with MCS cope and what gives them hope
when medical treatments, safe housing, relationships, career options
and self-esteem slip between their fingers?

These questions called to me to capture stories of people with
MCS who might provide the touchstones needed to survive this illness with a sense of self intact, to create a reservoir of stories to see
those with MCS through the dark passages we traverse. For my own
well-being I also needed to know: Who are these people who can be
incapacitated by one whiff of hair spray, fresh paint or after shave?
Deep down I feared that I might find them all to be eccentric or hopeless, because that is the image often portrayed by the media.

This quest took me from Louisiana to British Columbia and
points between to talk with people with MCS from all walks of life,
to see and experience the environments where they live, and to bring
together their powerful collective voice.

During each interview I stepped out of my role as a counselor,
called on my experience as a biographer and created a new role for
myself. As a fellow companion and seeker of hope and wisdom I
witnessed the following stories told to me in mutually beneficial
encounters. These stories of creativity and courage poured out to
me in the sacred spaces occupied by chemically-injured people, from
tiny oases in the desert to spacious urban homes custom-designed
to accommodate the chemically sensitive.

All individuals were asked the same basic questions: How has
MCS changed your life? How do you cope with isolation, fear,
stigma and loss? Where do you find hope? What, if any, positive
effects have you derived from these experiences? What would you

most like people to understand about you as a person with MCS? How do you hope others might be helped by hearing your story?

These narratives of men, women and children with MCS normalize the fear, loneliness, shame and loss that can torment those with this condition. They provide hope and encouragement desperately needed by others to persevere with MCS. Collectively, they can help others to avoid unnecessary chemical injuries, dispel some of the myths surrounding people with MCS, and bring greater insight and understanding to those who love, live with or work with someone who is chemically sensitive.

These stories represent people with different levels of impairment on the continuum of MCS, from moderate to severe, and are not intended to provide an accurate reflection of the demographics of the illness. The geographical locations reflect only my travel destinations.

Prevalence studies indicate that sixteen percent of the general U.S. population reports an unusual sensitivity to chemicals, and two percent have been diagnosed with MCS. Volumes could be filled with interviews from chemically sensitive people in any one state or region. For convenience I interviewed more people from the state of Washington, where I live, than from any other. However, to enjoy the benefits and richness of more diversity I also interviewed people from other parts of the U.S. and Canada, and one person from Belarus. Some of the people I interviewed were selected specifically because I knew of their accomplishments and assumed they must possess good coping strategies. Others were selected randomly according to places where I traveled, usually to visit my parents or other family members. I went to Santa Fe, New Mexico, and Snowflake, Arizona, specifically because I wanted to experience some of the places considered to be more environmentally safe than most parts of the country, and to talk with chemically sensitive people who have clustered there for that reason. My schedule allowed me to talk with more people in Santa Fe, some who lived there prior to developing MCS and others who moved there in desperation.

Newsletters and support group leaders proved to be fruitful resources for initial contacts, made by telephone prior to my trips. Each person I contacted expressed a desire to share with others the opportunity to give voice to the story of MCS, and volunteered referrals. The few who declined to be interviewed for personal reasons always offered some helpful bit of information or assistance of another kind. This unexpected enthusiasm and support nourished my spirit and kept my vision alive.

Originally I intended to eliminate any references to specific treatment or recovery protocols, because what works for one person can be harmful to others. Also, it is not uncommon for a relapse to follow a "recovery." The last thing I wanted was to publish false hopes, although some people with MCS do regain their health to various degrees. Once I began the interviews, however, I realized that it would tear away the heart and soul of the stories if I tried to make them fit a preconceived format. So, the essence of each story remains intact and some may include references to treatment modalities. Any theories, treatments, physicians or opinions mentioned do not necessarily reflect my own beliefs, are not published here as recommendations or endorsements, and should not be used to take the place of sound medical, psychological or legal advice tailored to the specific needs of individuals.

Like everyone, the people profiled in this volume are evolving. The narratives reflect their thoughts and experiences at the time of the interviews. Since then many have changed course in response to new research or personal growth, due to deteriorating or improved health, or all of the above. The themes and coping strategies they discuss, however, are timeless.

Observations

These stories describe some of the roads taken to solve the puzzle of illness caused by exposure to chemicals. For many the journey is long and involves a parade of doctors and misdiagnoses. Often MCS is discounted by health care professionals and others who doubt the validity of the illness. When the validity of an illness is discounted, the ill "suffer profound discord within their world," according to Kathy Charmaz in her book *Good Days, Bad Days: The Self in Chronic Illness and Time*. This discord can be heard in the collection of narratives in this volume.

What is remarkable to me is that those whose emotional, psychological and physical well-being is challenged daily by the environment possess such equanimity. Their stories are laced with love, depth, wisdom, growth, humor and creativity. Each of the interviewees with whom I met gifted me with a level of sincerity, warmth and respect that has become all too rare. Forced to simplify diet, activities and consumerism, many enjoy more balanced lifestyles than the average person. With lives pared down to only that which is most essential, they hear more clearly the voice within telling them what is meaningful. Many speak of a greater awareness of environmental issues and the interconnectedness of all people, and unexpected shifts toward altruistic values. Some respond to this with passion, others respond reluctantly out of a sense of obligation to the Earth and its inhabitants, or self-preservation.

The quality of life experienced by people with MCS is shaped, to a great extent, by the level of awareness of environmental health issues where they live and work. Some are recipients of workplace accommodations in accordance with the Americans with Disabilities Act; others are harassed and ostracized at work, or fired from their jobs. Some disabled by chemical exposures in the workplace receive workers' compensation; the majority of chemical-illness claims are denied. Some cities, schools and other institutions have adopted fragrance-free policies and Integrated Pest Management (IPM) programs to reduce chemical barriers and dangers in public places; others still resist despite all the prevalence studies and research indicating that MCS is a serious threat to public health.

The list of organizations and government agencies that recognize MCS is growing steadily. When a critical mass is reached, everyone will have access to safe housing, appropriate medical care, and chemical-free parks and public buildings; safe school environments will significantly reduce the incidence of learning disorders, behavior problems and chemically injured students and teachers. These are just a few of the possibilities, seemingly simple to achieve. Yet even these are still too few and far between; MCS is so hard to believe.

Industry stakeholders—including some physicians and researchers—and others with conflicts of interest have slowed both the research and the recognition of MCS. Human nature is on their side, because the reality of MCS can be difficult to accept even when you live with it. Most people trust that products on the market have been tested for human safety. Before the onset of MCS the thought never occurs to you that the ordinary products in your home or workplace could be affecting your health. Even after the connection is made we sometimes still deny the reality of those more sensitive than ourselves, until we reach that level. Don Paladin, one of the men I interviewed, describes this phenomenon well as he recalls an incident when, searching for a safe place for himself, he visited a chemically sensitive woman who sealed the air vents in her car to keep out fumes. Her efforts seemed excessive to him until years later when his own reactions to petrochemicals became so intolerable that he had to seal his car in a similar fashion in order to drive even a short distance.

Even more telling is an experience I had while talking on the phone with a woman who I didn't know, and who had been disabled by chemical exposures in her workplace. She was fired for missing work due to her illness, and had to take out a second mortgage in order to pay her medical bills. Her application for worker's compensation was denied. I spoke with her two days before the foreclosure on her house. With no money and no place to go, she was on the brink of joining the ranks of people who are homeless due to MCS. The gravity of her situation created in me an instant wave of denial. My fearful ego tried to convince me she'd been a loser all her life. The truth is, she'd been a hard-working, dependable employee at the same company for eighteen years, had lived in the same house for more than three decades.

Although I was shocked to see that kind of reaction in myself, it helped me to understand more deeply why the recognition of MCS is a slow and painful process.

What I've found is that most people with MCS struggle to remain employed and engaged in life, often at the expense of their health. Those who can no longer work held on as long as possible, and gave up their sources of income, esteem and identity only in desperation. I've found that homelessness can strike anyone with MCS, even someone with an abundance of financial resources. Several people whose stories appear in the following pages have experienced periods of homelessness because they couldn't find or couldn't afford environmentally safe housing, or both. One, Diane Hamilton, is a financially secure former chemist who resorted to sleeping first in an unfinished office building and later on a friend's porch when her own home was making her ill. Ann McCampbell, a medical doctor, talks about several critical periods when she had to sleep outside or in her car. Jennifer describes living outdoors in Colorado for most of four years. And Christina Jacobs, a former world-class athlete, has been living in her car for most of seven years.

Multiple chemical sensitivity involves coping with multiple losses. The loss of a safe home is one of the most devastating. Some other common losses touched upon in this collection of stories are self-esteem, relationships, mobility, careers, hobbies, access to public places and community events, transportation, tolerance to foods, and worship services. What I have tried to capture are the strength and grace that come from enduring and mourning these deep losses, and coming out the other side.

Because some people who self-disclose their vulnerability to chemicals become targets for hostility and violence, these narratives represent enormous acts of courage. When interviewing Katy Young, a single mother of two small children, I was deeply moved by her courage when she told me that after she received a death threat because of her work as an MCS activist, she tried to get out as much information as possible while she still could.

Among those I interviewed only two were bent toward politics, environmental issues or activism prior to their chemical injury. All formerly were consumers of products containing toxic chemicals. None of them are naïve enough to think it possible to eliminate all products containing toxic substances from society. Those who can, without serious consequences, still read newspapers or magazines printed with petroleum-based ink, use personal computers emitting radiation and plastic vapors, or still drive automobiles, for example. Reasonable goals include socially responsible use of potentially harmful products; adequate testing of chemicals on human safety; use of least-toxic products whenever possible; adoption of public policies to minimize chemical barriers in workplaces and on public property, and full disclosure of contents by manufacturers of all products, including so-called "inert" ingredients and those protected by trade secret laws. These steps would enable many people with MCS to remain employed and engaged in community activities, and would prevent many others from ever developing chemical injuries and environmental illnesses.

Everyone I interviewed was engaged in a process of self-healing, which means something different to each individual. To many it means that they have re-created a positive and productive life but would not expect to survive an extended exposure to toxic chemicals without serious consequences. Even those whose tolerance has improved dramatically are not inclined to revert back to using chemical-based products. Awakened to the effects of chemical exposures, it only makes sense to them to protect themselves, others, and the planet by using safe alternatives.

Most all of the people I interviewed would agree that stress and emotional turmoil can exacerbate MCS or any other illness. Many have increased their quality of life with MCS through emotional growth, stress management, spiritual deepening, or a combination of these. They all experience significant improvement in their health by avoiding chemical exposures.

I also witnessed among this population an extraordinary commitment to education, research and action aimed at understanding and preventing MCS. The dedication I observed was downright humbling. The majority of chemically injured people I've encountered are intelligent, resourceful, persevering, open and eager to share their wealth of experience and knowledge.

Understanding and confronting the issues related to chemicals and human health are among the most difficult endeavors one could pursue. One person extremely accomplished in this field was Cindy Duehring, a woman I did not have the privilege to meet. Cindy was a pre-med student in Seattle when she was severely poisoned by pesticides used by an exterminator to rid her apartment of fleas. She developed MCS so severe that she had to live in isolation in a specially filtered home built for her in North Dakota. There she founded the Environmental Access Research Network (EARN), an organization providing information on medical and legal issues related to toxics. In October 1997 it was announced in Stockholm, Sweden, that she was one of five people selected worldwide to receive the Right Livelihood Award for generating knowledge that can help others understand and combat the risks that toxic chemicals present to human life and health. This award is given to honor and support those offering practical and exemplary answers to the most urgent challenges facing us today. She lived and worked in isolation for twelve years before she died, of complications caused by her chemical injury, in 1999. Although she was unable to speak for the last two years of her life because, as a result of MCS, the sound of her own voice could trigger an audio-induced seizure, she continued her work in silence until several weeks before her death at age 36.

Inconsistencies, Frustrations and Accommodations

Accommodating a person with MCS can be as simple as opening a window. Or, it can be a frustrating exercise in patience and persistence, depending on the level of impairment, individual sensitivities, and type of environment. For example, someone with moderate MCS might be fine in a large group of people in a room with good ventilation and high ceilings, but unable to tolerate riding in a car with one person whose clothes were laundered with a scented detergent. A person's reactions can be immediate or delayed and they can vary according to the number of previous exposures in any given day or week, and other factors. These inconsistencies can baffle friends, family, coworkers and others who want to accommodate those with MCS. It can be confusing and frustrating to them when, after taking special precautions to be fragrance-free, the MCS person still experiences a chemical reaction. This happens frequently because most people do not realize how many of the products they use contain fragrances, and that some products labeled "unscented" actually contain a masking fragrance. It also can happen because many "fragrance-free" or "unscented" products contain other toxic chemicals. Or because our skin, hair and clothes pick up secondhand scents in our environment.

These individual differences and secondhand scents can make it difficult even for people who have MCS to meet the needs of each other. Faced with this challenge each time I conducted an interview for this book, I became aware of how difficult it must be for others to meet my requests for fragrance- and chemical-free encounters. As a precaution while traveling, I kept the clothes I would wear to interviews sealed in a plastic bag, protected from my other clothing, especially things I'd worn in airports and other places where fragrances can be intense. I also called ahead to inquire about any special requirements, and to let the person know that I would bring with me a change of clothes protected by a plastic bag from the secondhand scents I would encounter on my way to the appointment. I offered to change my clothes or take a shower, if necessary, upon arrival. As it turned out, the precautions I took led to safe encounters.

In addition to protecting others I was challenged by the difficulty of minimizing my own reactions to chemical exposures encountered in traveling: recirculated air on aircraft, hotel rooms and rental cars reeking from cleaning products, and public restrooms contaminated with toxic deodorizers, just to name a few. I tried to avoid early morning flights when other travelers' personal care products are fresh and strong, and I used a charcoal-filtered mask when necessary. But there were unavoidable consequences. On one trip, in the early stages of this project, I was in good shape when I boarded a plane to come home, and so ill by the time I arrived that it took me six weeks to recover. Another time, much later in the process, I had a severe chemical reaction on my way to Santa Fe. My head was pounding and I was so disoriented that I didn't know how I would be able to conduct interviews or find my way around town. With great effort I stripped the room of all the scented linens, replaced them with sheets and towels brought with me from home, took a shower to wash the secondhand fragrances off my skin, fortified my body with supplements and went to bed. This time I recovered by the next day. The bed and breakfast where I stayed in Santa Fe was fairly MCS-friendly, but I sometimes had to skip breakfast or a shower, or both, in order to avoid the drift of fragrances and other chemicals from the laundry room or other guests. Fortunately, I was able to stay in safe havens occupied by my parents in Michigan and on the Gulf Coast of Alabama on several trips, and drove to many of the interview appointments in fragrance-free cars provided by family members.

In return for my efforts I received the joys and blessings of a pilgrimage that began alone and ended with companions across the continent whose journeys toward wellness have provided me with powerful images of courage, hope and creativity. These images I now carry in spaces deep inside me once occupied by fear.

Whether you are an employer, landlord, friend, coworker, family member, health care professional or policymaker, a person who is mildly chemically sensitive or a universal reactor, may you find in these images an epiphany of your own.

To the MCS prophets—all reluctant at first—who have been given a great deal of responsibility for making Earth a safer place to live: Reclaim your power and voice. Tell your story. Open a door. Enjoy a moment of grace. Give thanks. Weep. Smile. Rage. Wear a mask. Breathe. You are part of a strong community scattered far and wide.

Midwest Stories

The tradition of storytelling is ageless and known to most cultures as an experience vital to the health of individuals, community and the environment.—Allison Cox and David Albert, the Healing Heart Project

Elizabeth Schuster
Detroit, Michigan

In December 1997, when the idea for this book was in its infancy, I saw Elizabeth Schuster's name and address on a list of new subscribers to an MCS newsletter. The listing caught my eye because she lives near my mother. Out of the blue I called Elizabeth to ask if I could interview her when I came to spend the holidays with my mother. She was the first person interviewed for this project, and I have since marveled at that good fortune. I found Elizabeth to be a woman of wonderful peace and grace. Hearing her story reconfirmed my belief in the healing power of stories, and strengthened my resolve to see this project to completion.

Elizabeth's ability to live well with MCS can be attributed in part to a supportive husband and an employer willing to make accommodations in her workplace. Since I interviewed her, a fragrance-free policy was adopted in her workplace, and environmental health issues have been considered in the planning of renovations in her department.

It is also crystal clear to me that Elizabeth's attitude also shapes her experience. She earned her doctorate after the onset of her illness. Now a professor of gerontology at a Midwestern university, she finds great satisfaction and joy in her work.

Elizabeth was a healthy child and has lived most of her life in Michigan. Except for two incidents when her joints swelled—once at age seven or eight and again in her teenage years—she had no signs of allergies until the birth of her first child. When I met her she was reactive to many foods and to most vitamins, herbal supplements and medications in addition to chemicals.

Elizabeth's reactions to chemical exposures can be so severe

19

that she sometimes must use oxygen to cope. Among the products troublesome to her is clothing. Because she reacts to chemicals used to treat fabrics, she is unable to wear most new or used clothing, even after many washings.

Since I first interviewed Elizabeth I have had the pleasure of visiting with her several times when I was in the Midwest. When I decided to include in my book an interview with a family member of a person with MCS, I asked her husband, Curt, because I knew they enjoyed a strong and healthy relationship. They have two children—a teenaged son and a married daughter.

It's not this illness that's determining how I live. I've never been happier. I've never been more whole. I've never been as peaceful or as calm as I am at this moment. And I just assume it will become more so. Even if my outer world becomes more compressed and limited, my inner world, at the same time, is expanding. This is a time of real growth and change and insight for me.

That's not to say there aren't times when I just want to give it up. There have been times that have been pure hell.

The hardest thing for me in having a problem that has not been recognized by the medical community is to have the onus placed on the person who is not well, to almost be in a defensive position. I am someone who understands persons wanting proof, evidence, a scientific orientation. I want to say, Just hook me up to an MRI or CAT scan and expose me to perfume and watch what happens to my brain!

Probably the area that has changed the most in my life is letting go of what is "normal," letting go of the idea that something is "wrong" if I can't live my life the way it used to be, not being able to go places and do things. The hardest thing is to remember how it was before, all the things that I could do. I remember the realization—when I bought a new piece of clothing and put it on and started getting high from it—that I can't wear new clothes anymore. I can't go with my husband to his parents' house. I cannot ever buy a new car again. I can never dry clean anything. I cannot swim in pools again. My house is desperately in need of paint and new carpet, but that is out of the question. It's very hard to travel or to go to hotels.

Most people just get in the car and go to a movie or a restaurant or wherever. The first thing in my mind is, Is it safe? Is there going to be someone next to me loaded with perfume? The world has changed that way.

My energies are much more into other aspects of my life, but there are times when I feel obligated to enlighten and educate others, to help people understand, not just for myself. When I got this I didn't want to play that role. I don't want to be the one they're talking about twenty, thirty, fifty years from now when they're writing in textbooks about this, that "these people were showing us what was

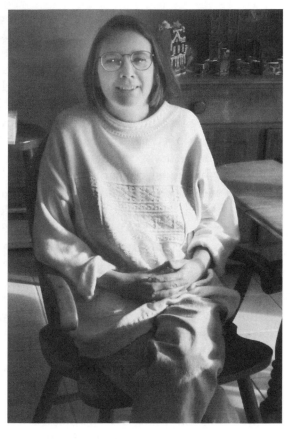

happening to the air, to the water." I'd much rather go to the store and buy a bucket of paint and paint this house, I'm so tired of the dirty marks on the wall! I don't want to have to wear clothes that are spotted, or have to worry about spilling on them because I know it's the only sweater I can still wear. But my friends and family and people I work with read the same information, and pretty much come at it the same way (as the mainstream medical community), so what I've had to do is educate them, enlighten them. My daughter is in cosmetology! She still forgets and wears something, and I just say I can't be around her right now. We deal with it with humor.

At work, at the start of every class I teach, I pass out literature and a memo to my students: "Please do not wear perfume. This will help me to concentrate and be much more with it during teaching." When I have to bring it up people say: "You know, I just went into a room," or, "I just bought a new car, and I got the worst headache!"

People start to connect, but there's always "I'm not as bad as *you*—thank God!"

Looking back on my life, there probably were other symptoms when I was younger but I didn't make the connection. After my first child was born I was real tired and had some tests done. They thought I was anemic because my iron level was low, but even the hematologists said it was not low enough to be causing my fatigue. I also developed food allergies I'd never had before.

Nine years ago when we moved to our first house, I painted and we had extensive work done in the bathroom, tiling and things. Then we had wall-to-wall carpeting put in—and something happened. It was such a dramatic effect, unlike I'd ever had before. Not just feeling tired, but disoriented. I lost my glasses—never found them. Things like that. The smell of the carpet was so strong, and I felt better when I went outside. We tore out the carpet and had new floors put in, and my life just went on normally. We continued to use the same cleaning products and everything. Everything seemed fine, but I'm sure the chemicals were slowly affecting me even though I could still tolerate a lot of things I can't now.

Things finally started clicking into place, like a light going on, when we moved into our present house, five years ago. That was probably one of the most traumatic experiences of my life. I'd come in the house and sat here and talked and seemed okay. But when we moved in, the pain in my head was excruciating. It was the start of a whole year of hell, trying to get this house safe and the real-ization of what I'd done—bought a place that made me ill. You've signed all the papers and spent thousands of dollars, there's no way out. I guess that's the frightening feeling, that there's no way out. That's when I just started realizing what was going on with chem-icals, and from there it just escalated, it just kept going.

I was on oxygen for the first year here, and I had to wear a mask at times. I was worried about the kids and how they'd feel about Mom being on oxygen. But it wasn't like I was dying. I was still going to work and making dinner, so it wasn't that big of a deal to them.

When I'm sitting in a chair with an oxygen tank, just trying to recover, those are the hardest times for my husband, I think. For him the anger comes from not being able to do anything about it. If he can do something—anything—it helps him to get it out. He just wants to help me to be well, and he can't.

Each time I experience a major loss or setback from this illness, something that I know is going to cause major changes in my life, the grieving process goes really deep. I led bereavement support groups for six years, so I know something about the grief process, and you can't stop it. To do so is to halt the process momentarily because you're going to go back in, eventually. There are times when I still resist. At those times there's a voice, far down, that is assuring me that it's going to be okay again.

Sometimes I just let it happen, not try to resist. I just say, okay, there's gonna be the blues. I think it's human nature, when a crisis hits, to want to live like an animal and go burrow in for a while, at some point. I have to do this sometimes. That's when I bring in the support systems, when it gets that bad. I have my husband, my family, and, at times, a therapist. It helps just to talk about it. For me, being able to tell my story over and over again, what happened and how it happened, I think that's a very natural need, to get it out of the mind, to get it spoken, for someone else to understand and to show me some kind of empathy. The story about the house and moving in was one I told very frequently when it first happened.

When people are going through the grief process, just about anything they feel is normal. With this illness, a lot of the feelings you have may be feelings you've never had before because you've never experienced that stage of grief. I think that's the most important thing for people to know, that you might feel like an alien inside. That's part of it.

One of the times I grieved most was when they remodeled the building where I had worked. I knew I was going to have a problem, but I didn't know to what extent. I ended up having to move my office to another building for two years. Except for a couple of people, my colleagues didn't know about my problem until that happened. I felt exposed when they learned I wasn't just like them. I had to take on an extra level of strength. For the most part they were caring. When we had meetings they came to my office. For them it was no problem. My whole life was changing.

It's tempting to hold onto what was, wanting things to be the way they were even though they might not have been that great. What I'm working on now is the definition of what is "okay." That's tough work. Hard work. Heart work.

There have been times when I just wanted to give up. I went through a period, during the first few years when I realized what was happening, and there was one loss after the next, when I thought I should leave because I was ruining my family's life. They can't live normal lives, and they have to live in a house like this. I thought that if I died my husband could marry another woman and he could paint the house, put in carpet, buy a new car, all of it. But that's just nonsense. The connection between my husband and me is so much more important than material possessions. I guess if he were someone whose identity was all wrapped up in his living environment or what kind of car he drove, then we'd have a lot of trouble. He has had to let go. There were hard times that would stress any relationship.

Coping has a lot to do with your family and how they respond. The relationships that preceded the illness are important. That's true of any crisis, but with this, I think, it becomes tantamount because the family has to change. This is different than cancer, for example, because this is all pervasive. You can't go anywhere without there being a risk of being affected.

I'm thankful for the external supports that I have, but all the external supports in the world—love and kindness and understanding—won't help if it doesn't come from within. It's the internal supports that are critical.

I've been meditating since I was twenty. A lot of meditation is about letting go, and awareness, and understanding. The people who seem to be able to move through chronic situations with some sense of grace and integrity are those who willingly go within and attempt to understand what's going on in all ways, emotionally, physically, psychologically, spiritually. Meditation has moved me along that path. It has accelerated. My husband and I are moving into practicing more insightful meditation, reading much more about Buddhist philosophy. Buddhism is much more an exploration of one's internal world, understanding the experience of what it is to be alive, being really aware and conscious, loving one's self, and forgiving. It's so easy to come down so hard on yourself.

That kind of awareness, that centeredness, allows me to move away from being reactive to being much more proactive. If a chemical swings me out of balance, I focus on bringing my energy back into balance. The amount of energy or inner strength I need to do that is tremendous. It's a real learning experience that takes awareness. It's empowering to look at this as a way to learn something about myself.

Part of this internal work is letting go of the false belief that we really have a whole lot of control, and to stay focused in the moment, right here, without projecting into what might happen. To purely experience whatever happens as it happens, not before and not after.

What I'm trying to figure out is, what happens if I get cognitively impaired and I'm attempting to be mindful? Am I really in this internal work for the long ride, or only as long as things are okay? If I cross over a line and I cannot get back, then what do I do? Just saying that, I can feel the fear. It's like a child's fear and when it comes up I'm not in control anymore. I won't know until that happens, if it does happen. I don't dwell on that, because I don't know.

A couple of weeks ago at work I got hit with one of the worst kinds of chemicals for me. It was a chemical they used to treat a floor, and I didn't know it was there when I walked in. I had a panic-type reaction because it was one of those chemicals that I can feel moving into my brain and grabbing on, and it won't let go. One that affects me for three, four, five days, even with oxygen and taking hot baths. Those chemicals tend to cause personality changes in me. I lose part of who I am briefly. I lose the ability to connect, and I can become mean. I'm sure that's a combination of the chemical and being scared. It's a frightening thing when I get hit with that kind of a chemical, which, thank God, isn't often. That's when I get scared. For me the thing that works best is hard-core exercise. I get on the exercise bike and get the blood going up to the brain. I think it just cleanses me. Thankfully, I've recovered every time.

Only a couple of my friends or anyone at work has seen me when I'm hit like that. Usually I operate normally. It's almost like acting. I'm so used to having my brain get kind of swollen if I get hit by perfume or something, and I know that I'm going to get back to normal within a matter of minutes or hours or even a day after the person leaves. But when I get hit with the worst stuff, it's like I give up. The chemical takes such a hold on me I almost give in to it. I can't function anymore, and I'm not sure I'm going to get back.

How I experience that and how others experience that with me will have a great deal to do with the work that I do inside myself. What I do in my mind will have a tremendous influence on whatever happens. I might not be able to manipulate my environment but I can sure do a lot with my inner world while I still have the functioning. I do have a choice. Remaining calm and at peace even when the whole world seems to be in chaos, that's a choice I'm learning to make. I don't know if I would be growing in this way if I wasn't coping with MCS. Not at this pace. It might be that I need to move at this pace. I don't know how fast my chemical sensitivity is accelerating. But right now I'm able to be okay. And I take full responsibility for keeping myself healthy and as active and happy and content as possible because no one else is going to do it for me.

I eat healthfully—I always have, but even more so now. My life-style is really healthy in all ways. In the winter I'm on the exercise bike four times a week, pretty much hard-core riding for forty-five minutes. When the weather is good I walk four or five miles, or I ride my bike six, seven miles, two or three times a week. I do yoga, and have for twenty-five years. If I'm keeping my body really strong, it's not just exercising to stay in shape physically, it's my whole being.

I really hope that both my kids are healthy lifelong. God forbid if they have to go through this, but you never know. They have their own paths. Neither of them are showing any problems with the environment, that I know of. And they're coming from a home and a life of great strength. They're going to be way ahead of me.

My husband and I both have a real love of nature. We do a lot of skiing, walking, hiking, working in the garden. I spend a lot of time with my family. We play games and read and cook together, get videos. There is one movie theater where I can go. I tend to go off-hours, and if somebody wearing perfume sits next to me, I just get up and move. I don't go the first day of a movie when it's packed.

I have not worn masks out in public because of the stigma. If I'm at a concert or some other public event, I sit with a handkerchief or a scarf over my nose. I'll wear a mask in the car sometimes, and I have an oxygen tank in the car.

Being a professor, a lot of time and energy is given to teaching, reading papers, writing, researching. Thankfully, my work is my joy. Recently I flew to Washington, D. C., to make a presentation. It was such a joy because the presentation was well received, the hotel was one of the safest places I've ever been, and I was able to fly without any problems. I felt like I used to feel before I had this illness. So I'm hoping travel will become more of a possibility.

Even though my thinking is not as sharp and clear, my ability to reason and to communicate and understand is probably deeper and broader than ever. Who knows, I could have tissue damage in my brain from the swelling and numbness caused by chemicals, but I am doing more cognitive and intellectual work than I ever have in my life. It's a different kind of thinking.

As I became more and more sensitive over the last five or six years, I was seeing a therapist. That helped, just to talk about it with the therapist and my husband and my family. There's only one person out of my group of friends who I really feel understands. It's still hard for people who don't have this to understand. It's only when times are really bad, which is infrequent, that it's an issue. Most of my friends don't wear perfume, and no one at work wears perfume anymore. Every year I put out a memo at the beginning of the year saying: "Thank you so much for your kindness and thoughtfulness and your awareness of my sensitivities to fragrances." People really appreciate it. They want to do whatever will work. And I operate normally.

When I go to meetings or get asked to go somewhere, I kind of brace myself before I walk in the door. When I get in and see it's safe, then I can be there as I was before this happened, and talk as usual. I've gotten more bold about asking people if they've painted or put in new carpeting. Then I have to be ready for the questions. I kind of set myself up doing that. But I'd rather do that than walk in and say, "I can't be here"—which I've had to do. Most people know about it now, they know right away we're going to have to move. We've gotten used to socializing with all of these issues.

Everyone has to decide for themselves what makes life meaningful and worth living. For me, it is to practice loving. I think that's why we're here. As human beings we have the capacity to love in all ways. I think that's what brings great meaning and joy, even when you lose total mental abilities. It's much more than the ability to emote. I think as long as there is life, there is love. Life is love. This moment is what you have, so do with it what brings you great meaning.

Those of us with MCS need to treat ourselves as we would treat a young child with this illness, with love and compassion. We tend to be really hard on ourselves. We need to envision the most loving person we've ever known or heard of, to look into that person's eyes with total love and to feel that for ourselves. Practicing forgiveness is the most important thing, forgiveness of ourselves and others. Truly forgive. I think that a combination of letting go and forgiveness is the best that any of us can do.

Another important thing is to accept others' care for us. Our society is overly involved with individuality and autonomy and independence. And I'm all for that. We all want to be independent and able to take care of ourselves. But we have a really tough time accepting care and, therefore, we have a tough time caring for ourselves. I'm seriously thinking about writing an article titled "What's Wrong with Dependency?"

There are many things in the world one could choose to feel doom and gloom about. The real challenge is to look upon all the world with eyes of empathy and compassion for everyone who is suffering. Just about every soul in this world is suffering for one reason or another, I think. Right now I just happen to have a condition that's a little odd.

Lynn Lawson
Evanston, Illinois

Lynn Lawson moves in one direction only: forward. Adversity and closed doors don't deter her. The book she wrote, Staying Well in a Toxic World, *was published after forty-five rejections, and now is in its third printing. Lynn is a leader of the Chicago-area MCS support group; editor of* CanaryNews, *a newsletter with subscribers nationwide; a founder of the National Coalition for the Chemically Injured; and a member of Alliance for Democracy, a political group seeking increased social responsibility from corporations. She never misses an opportunity to educate or influence any potential audience, through contacts with administrators, writers, politicians, educators and others.*

Lynn lived and worked with migraine and other headaches for more than forty years. At age sixty she retired, hoping that that might bring her some relief. When that didn't help, she finally followed through with a referral to Dr. Theron Randolph, known as the founder of modern environmental medicine. Under his care Lynn finally reclaimed her health and began her second career, as an MCS educator and advocate.

Lynn believes the success of her recovery is due, in part, to the quality of her early life. Raised in Wisconsin at a time when farmers put manure, not synthetic chemicals, on their fields, she ate only organic foods because that was all there was. Her mother, a physiotherapist in World War I and keenly interested in health, raised her as a vegetarian, although she now eats meats. Lynn describes her mother as a forerunner of the holistic practitioner.

Now in her seventies, Lynn addresses her concerns regarding the lack of safe retirement homes and nursing facilities for elderly people with MCS who are unable to continue living in their own homes.

Our conversation took place at O'Hare International Airport, where Lynn came to meet me during a brief layover.

During the forty-plus years that I was increasingly sick with headaches, I thought I had this incurable disease called migraines. But after a few months of avoiding the chemicals and foods that I tested positive to, my headaches greatly diminished. I finally knew what most other people must feel like most of the time. That was a turning point in my life.

At the age of twelve or thirteen I had my first migraine aura. The aura started with a blank spot in the middle of my vision, and gradually became flickering zigzag lights that covered about half my vision by the end of the episode. They lasted half an hour and were followed by a characteristic kind of head pain. I didn't know what they were; I thought I must be going blind. My mother rarely took me to doctors, and she never took me to a doctor about this, that I can recall. They may have been connected with hormones, the onset of menstruation.

My *big* problem with headaches, however, started after I graduated from Beloit College in 1946. I was a chemistry major, with a double major in English. I remember the awful smells in the chemistry building.

My first job out of college was at the Argonne National Laboratory, near Chicago, from 1946 to 1954. My work took me into

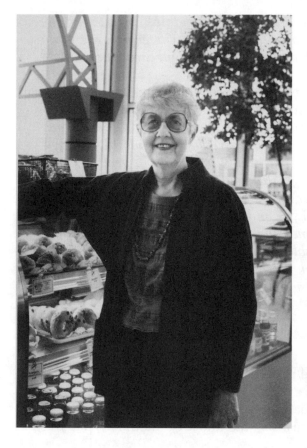

the library of the University of Chicago's chemistry department, where I was hit with more smells. Eventually I was assigned to an office in the middle of Argonne's chem lab, where I was surrounded by chemicals. I started getting "common" migraines, where you have a headache but no aura. Over the next forty years, these headaches became increasingly frequent and increasingly severe.

Later I worked at the Art Institute of Chicago, where the walls were painted for every new exhibit. In the 1970s I started working in new buildings, tightly built, with sealed windows and wall-to-wall carpeting. That's when I really began to get worse, with non-aura, all-over-sick headaches two and three days a week. I'd wake up early with a severe headache, and I'd take aspirin with milk—which, I later learned, only added to my misery. Usually this didn't work; I'd feel worse and worse during the day.

I knew that tobacco smoke bothered me and I didn't like perfumes, and I didn't like the deodorant or soap that some of my clients used. But I didn't know why.

In 1971 my internist told me about Dr. Randolph and his environmental unit, where I would be fasted for about four days and then tested for foods and chemicals. I couldn't face going into the unit because I knew that whenever I missed even one meal, I would get a headache so terrible that my head would hurt even on the softest pillow. Later I learned that this was because I was missing my "fix"—my morning milk and other foods I was dependent on or addicted to. Since I didn't know this was the cause, I didn't go. I suffered for fifteen more years.

In 1985 I retired at the age of sixty. I thought that stress might be causing my headaches, and that if I quit work I might get better. During that first year of retirement my husband and I had walls painted in our house, and I got sick from the paint. I became more active in our church, and I'd get a headache the day after going there. So I quit going to church and I stopped being active. I dreaded social occasions. People say this is agoraphobia, but I knew it was because I got sick everywhere. I wasn't getting any better at all.

After a year of this I went to my internist and said, "I'm desperate, tell me more about your Dr. Randolph." He gave me the phone number of Dr. Randolph's clinic and said, "I wouldn't wait any longer; he's not getting any younger." Dr. Randolph was almost eighty then.

When I went to him, it was a real eye-opener. I saw what happened to other people in the testing room and I saw what happened to me. I learned that I had both food sensitivities and chemical sensitivities.

At the end of my testing I was put on a strict avoidance and rotational diet, and my reaction was overwhelming. Suddenly I was terribly sick from withdrawal, with an excruciating headache for two days.

The diagnosis meant many changes. We had our gas kitchen stove removed and an electric stove put in. There was a lot to do to find new, safer products. I made out a two-week chart to keep track of everything I could eat, trying to cut it down to one or two foods per meal so that I could pinpoint and control my food sensitivities. It was hard because I didn't know anybody else who had this problem. I joined a local support group as soon as I found out about it, and that was a real blessing.

Over the next year I gradually got better. I was delighted that everything I learned about and did was finally relieving my headaches. But there were many losses.

There were so many foods that I "lost," and we gave up going to plays, movies, and the opera, and eating out. But the biggest loss for me was my best friend.

When my husband and I were at her house soon after I was diagnosed, I realized that her detergent was bothering me, so I called her the next day and told her about it. I thought she would be receptive because she was interested in the environment. Later she called and said she wanted to come over to talk. Her husband dropped her off and we had what my husband and I refer to as "the kitchen scene." She told me she thought that my illness was psychological and that I needed to see a psychiatrist. I said, "Let me give you Dr. Randolph's book [*An Alternative Approach to Allergies*]." She took it, and two days later she called and said she didn't believe it.

I was very disappointed, and we saw each other less often for a while. But the real break came later when she said, "I don't want to hear any more about your chemical dependence." I said, "Chemical *dependence*! What do you mean? It's not chemical *dependence*, it's just the opposite!" She said that she didn't want to hear anything more about it, and that we shouldn't see each other for a while. That was the final break.

When she hung up I screamed and screamed and cried and cried. The grief and anger—oh, my God. That was devastating. I have no brothers or sisters, and she was like a sister to me. I thought it was a lifelong relationship, and I lost her.

What do I do with my anger? Be active on behalf of people with environmentally related illnesses, such as multiple chemical sensitivities. I wrote my book for that reason. My book is the single most important thing I have accomplished in my entire life. I wrote it to try to validate the illness for people who know they have it, and to warn the people who don't know they have it. I wrote it to help people.

In 1991 I became coordinator of the support group; I am now a PR chair and editor of its newsletter. I've done national radio talk shows. I write letters. That's the way I cope. There's hardly a day when I don't do something for people with environmental illness and MCS. I really function as a servant, serving people. I never wanted to be a social worker, but I find I'm often functioning as one, albeit untrained. EI/MCS is an illness often ignored or attacked as fraudulent. Many of its victims fall into society's cracks, without adequate recognition or support.

I tell the stunned, desperate people who call me that there is hope. I've gotten better and I know other people who've gotten better; there's a good chance that they'll get better if they do what's necessary. Avoidance is still the best therapy.

I'm a clearinghouse of information. I help people with information about doctors, about products. I have piles and piles of information. People who've read my book, or people in the support group or prospective members contact me. I spend a lot of time sending information to people, as well as just listening. At times I'm overwhelmed with all I have to do; sometimes it's really more than I can handle. I don't think I could have done what I have without my husband; he has always been supportive. Also, I have made a lot of wonderful new friends.

The only thing that relieves my anxiety is getting things done. But I do manage to take care of myself and do what I need to do to stay well—eating organic, unprocessed foods and obtaining special foods, supplements and other products from catalogs.

I'd like to see more people becoming active writing letters, because I think that does help. I sent forty copies of my book to famous people—legislators, senators, celebrities, media people. In my cover letter I focused on the Gulf War Syndrome, which many of us see as a variation of EI/MCS.

I see signs that there is more acceptance. There are more books out. In our church, the son of a friend in our support group won, in an auction, the chance to pick the subject for a sermon, and he picked multiple chemical sensitivities. The minister gave the sermon, and a committee was established to make the church more accessible to people with MCS. Now I can get a "Fragrance Free" sign to hang on the back row when I attend.

Full acceptance may never come, because of intense industry resistance, but there will be more acceptance when a celebrity who has the illness is properly diagnosed.

I'd like to see people get involved with a new grassroots group that my husband and I have joined, the Alliance for Democracy. It's a growing national group with five thousand members who are trying to make corporations more accountable. State-granted charters can be revoked—and have been in the past—if corporations are not functioning in the public interest. A good sign is that this group asked people to come unfragranced to their organizational meeting in Texas. Can you imagine any political party asking people not to wear fragrances? I couldn't believe it!

What am I afraid of? I'm really afraid of getting old because I don't know how I'll take care of myself. Where am I going to go? I don't want to enter a nursing or retirement home because of all the unsafe products people use there. So my husband and I plan to go on living in our house, retrofitting it where needed. We are lucky to have recently located an eldercare case manager who is also chemically sensitive.

My goals are to keep distributing my book, to continue building up the support group, and to keep on writing the newsletter. I can't do these things forever. Because I have macular degeneration, I may lose my eyesight, in which case I will have to stop. And that will be very frustrating.

At this point I don't have to give up much, but I still take precautions. When we go to concerts or movies, I hold a charcoal filter tight to my nose. When we travel, I take my own bedding and an air purifier, even to Europe. I can go for months without getting a headache. When I do get one, it's mild—nothing like having severe ones two or three days a week. Unlike many, I'm able to lead a fairly normal life. I'm very fortunate.

Nicholas Elijah Weiss
Toledo, Ohio

Nicholas Weiss, nine when interviewed, had difficulty sleeping and needed to be walked constantly as an infant. His symptoms worsened as he grew. He experienced learning and behavioral problems in school, temper tantrums, and frequent headaches. He made suicidal statements such as "I'm so angry I want to kill myself," and "I'm so stupid I want to kill myself." Traditional testing showed no abnormalities. When his food and chemical sensitivities finally were identified and he avoided these triggers, his self-esteem, school performance and behavior improved dramatically. In the fifth grade he made the honor roll. After meeting with him, I can understand why his mother now describes him as "a charming individual."

Nicholas enjoys basketball, football and hockey; riding his bike and reading Goosebumps and other stories. His favorite subjects in school are science and social studies.

I never got all my work done. I couldn't listen well and I couldn't learn. I kept telling myself, "I have to get this stuff done!" I didn't know what was going on.

After I started eating the food I'm supposed to eat I started feeling better, and I do a lot better in school.

Twenty-eight allergies, that's how many I have. I can hardly name them all.

When I was tested for my allergies I thought: Oh, I hope I don't have to give up ice cream! I hope I don't have to give up bread! I hope I don't have to give up this and that. Well, it turned out to be all of that. I had to give it all up. No sugar. No chocolate. No milk. Can't have ice cream. Can't have corn. Can't have wheat.

I'm also allergic to mold, and dust, and formaldehyde. Sometimes when I walk into a mall I get a headache and my nose starts running. I can smell the formaldehyde. If I use strong shampoos my ears get real red and hot and they stay like that for a couple of hours, and I don't feel well. And if I smell perfume I get a headache real bad and it hurts my stomach. At school I plug my nose when the teachers walk by with perfume on. They clean the floor with stuff that I'm allergic to, so my head hurts all day. But they have to do that to keep their job.

When the pollen is out, that really bothers me. When I go outside I get *big* headaches and my ears turn red and burn. Sometimes I just go out and try to forget about it, and sometimes I don't go outside.

I get scared when I go outside and ride my bike real fast and run into flowers where there's bees. I'm allergic to bees. If I got stung my throat would close up and I couldn't breathe and I'd get real big hives. I could die from it.

Once I ran over a bee and it was still alive and it chased me, but I turned a corner and lost it. And one time I was in the basement and a dead bee dropped from the ceiling. It got caught in my shirt and I went upstairs and sat on the couch, and I just barely put my back against the couch and I jumped up and started screaming. When bees are dead they can still sting you, and I had to go to the hospital.

I take special foods to school to eat. Older kids used to tease me. They'd say, "That's disgusting!" Sometimes they'd push me, and

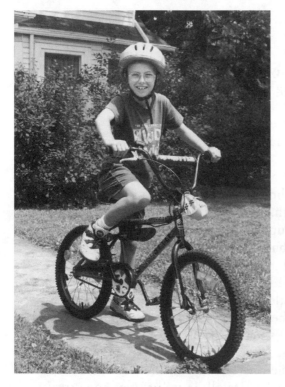

I'd just walk away. After I told on them a couple million times, they stopped. Now they don't tease me. A lot of other people bring their own food to school, too, so I don't feel weird.

When I go to a friend's house, sometimes my mom will pack a lunch for me. Or, if there's spaghetti I'll just pick out the noodles without trying to make it look disgusting, and I just eat the sauce. If they have hot dogs, I just cover it with mustard and ketchup and I don't eat the bun. It's sort of hard because I like hot dogs with a bun, but that gives me a headache. Hot dogs without the bun give me a headache, too.

Sometimes I don't feel like eating the stuff I can eat. So I just don't eat, or I ask my mom or grandma to make me something special. Grandma makes good pizza without wheat. It falls apart and the stuff on top won't stick to it, but I don't mind, I just eat it with my fork or spoon. At home I can eat a rice cake with peanut butter, or something like that.

I wish I could eat food that other people eat. Sometimes, like once a month, I'm allowed to eat something I'm not supposed to.

I would tell other kids who have allergies to stay on their diet for a couple of years, then they might be able to eat others things once a month or so, like me. And try not to use cleaning liquids and things like that, and to keep their room clean.

If people who read my story have a child or niece with allergies, maybe they'll understand more and not just say it's nothing.

Southwest Stories

As a prevention tool, storytelling is a time-tested craft that can tackle the challenges confronting our culture. Because story has proven throughout time to be a vehicle for the mind to make sense of the world, it has been used by humankind through the centuries as a means of transmitting important cultural, sociological and moral information from one generation to the next.—Allison Cox, storyteller

Ann McCampbell
Santa Fe, New Mexico

Ann McCampbell, M.D., is a graduate of the UCLA Medical School and became a licensed physician in California in 1979. She completed an internship in internal medicine in Santa Barbara, and practiced in the field of women's health for five years at the University of California Santa Barbara Student Health Center, and at Kaiser Permanente in the San Francisco Bay Area. Off-hours she played drums in a rock and roll band, and played competitive beach volleyball.

In one week in 1989 Ann's health deteriorated rapidly from MCS. Her medical career had abruptly ended nine months earlier when she sustained a back injury. She went from living an active, athletic life to living in the backseat of her Chevy Impala. Although her medical license is current she is still unable to practice medicine due to severe physical limitations.

Known far and wide for her success as an MCS activist and educator, Ann moved to New Mexico in the early 1990s in search of a safer house and environment. Santa Fe hasn't been the same since her arrival. She recently was recognized by leaders of the city for her contributions to the community. She was one of the founders of the Healthy Housing Coalition of New Mexico, a non-profit organization providing information on MCS and New Mexico, and tips for creating safe housing.

Ann, forty-nine when interviewed, described herself to me as an easygoing person with an intense core, a diplomatic type who can relate well to all kinds of people. I found this description to fit her to a "T," and would add to that other endearing and admirable qualities. She is intelligent, persevering, spontaneous and genuine.

A certain vulnerability comes across from her, coupled with a strength and a sense of self that comes from enduring a deep loss or tragedy. She's a bit of a maverick, playful, sometimes hilarious, most of the time incredibly serious.

Ann now lives eighteen miles out of town in the desert. Because her roommate is too ill with MCS to risk exposure to other people, Ann and I rendezvoused in the parking lot of the Wild Oats store, a popular meeting place for people with MCS in Santa Fe. From there I followed her to the home of one of her friends, where Ann put on her respirator in the parking lot to get her safely past the laundry area and into her friend's apartment. Sitting in the sun on the patio, she told to me the following story.

I'm pretty thrilled to still be alive. Within one week, in 1989, my life changed forever. Since then there have been times when I've had to really work to stay alive.

During the time I was working as a physician for Kaiser Permanente in the Bay Area, I lifted a box and protruded a disk in my back and developed severe bilateral sciatica. Most people with this condition would do a few exercises and be in pretty good shape in a month, and with additional conditioning they'd be a hundred percent better in six months to a year. My back didn't behave normally. Anything that was supposed to help only made it worse.

Not long after that, I was at work when I stood up and my whole leg was numb and couldn't hold my weight. I limped out, and that was my last day of work. I had to lie flat on my back for the next several years. Today my back is finally strong enough that I can sit for a while, but even taking a blood pressure would be difficult and painful for me.

In the beginning I thought I had a back problem that wasn't healing properly, and I didn't understand why, other than I wasn't getting proper nutrition. I had been having severe digestion problems for several years. All I was able to eat was fish and a few vegetables. I was in search of another protein source that I could tolerate. I tried a little chicken broth, and that didn't work. I tried frog legs, and that didn't work. Quail eggs didn't work. Finally I tried a hypoallergenic protein powder and had the worst food reaction of my life. My heart started racing like I was injected with adrenaline. I couldn't sleep. My stomach was in knots. I felt nauseated. All I could eat after that was a little bit of broccoli, carrots and purple cabbage, and that came right through me unchanged. I was really scared.

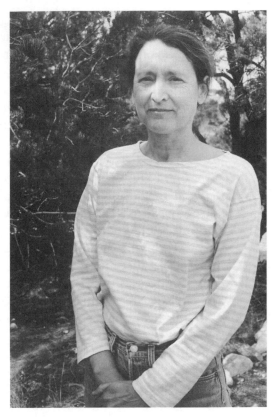

Over a very short period of time—a few days—I felt my sense of smell increase by about twenty-fold. I became reactive to what felt like every molecule that came by. I even had to cover the metal buttons on my jacket, because I reacted to them. I couldn't stay in my home because of mold and pesticides inside. But I had no place to go. So I threw a foam pad outside on the ground, and just lay there. My back was so bad at that time that I had to lie down all the time. I could stand to be up ten or fifteen minutes a couple of times a day, just long enough to go inside, steam some vegetables and get back outside to lie down and eat. That was so difficult for me, to be unable to move. I'd always been such a physical person, and here I was not even able to cry because I couldn't hold that much tension in my body without hurting my back more.

That summer of 1989, from May until October, was the most miserable, unbelievable experience of my life. I didn't know what was going on. I couldn't believe something so horrible could be happening to me, and that my life had turned to this. It was like being in a strange episode of *The Twilight Zone*.

I call that summer of 1989 my "Vietnam" period, because the level of trauma I experienced was like living in a war zone. It was like constantly walking over land mines. And sniper fire could happen anytime.

My thyroid function went down to nothing. I couldn't believe

I was still breathing. I knew I had to get supplemented with thyroid hormone, and I couldn't imagine what was going to work. I couldn't see how I was going to pull out of it. Death seemed imminent.

All of my medical knowledge was of no use. I knew this was way beyond medical knowledge. I knew that if *I* didn't know what was wrong, there weren't going to be many doctors who did. I didn't have faith that some doctor was going to be able to fix me.

I went to see an endocrinologist. It was difficult because I had to protect myself from exposures to fragrances while I was there, even though I knew the doctor thought I was crazy and people were sneering at me. I said to this doctor, "Maybe I need a GI workup, because my gut isn't working and I can't eat." He said, "Your gut is working fine. What you need is to see a psychiatrist!"

Even though I didn't agree with that, I remembered from my training that sometimes when people with irritable bowel syndrome took antidepressants for some other reason, the irritable bowel improved. So, I was thinking that if my gut problem was a neurological one, it might respond to a psychoactive agent. So I did go to see a psychiatrist. I told him my whole story and said, "What do you think?" He said, "The diagnosis is obvious, it's anorexia." I said, "Yes, but not anorexia nervosa. Anorexia just means you're not eating, and I'm not eating because I can't tolerate the food." We obviously disagreed on that. He recommended I take Prozac, but when he said two of the side effects were anorexia and nausea, I said, "I really don't think that is going to help." Then I got up and left.

Although I didn't know what was happening to me at the time I was hit with this illness, I wasn't totally clueless about MCS. I had friends with environmental illness, but I had no idea of the gravity or the breadth of the whole thing. One woman couldn't come into my home because of mold in it. Another one mentioned problems she'd had at work when the parking lot was resurfaced, and when coworkers wore perfume. But no one had told me that my laundry soap, or bleach, or body soaps could make me ill. The people I knew with MCS could still function in the world. I had it about as bad as it gets.

In the beginning, when I was reacting to so many things, I really couldn't sort it all out. But I found a fact sheet on safe products that someone had given to me, and I asked somebody to buy me the things on the list, trusting that would help. I knew there were environmental doctors, and I hung to the hope that one of them would be able to help me. Unfortunately, I learned that physicians can be treated differently than other patients, there can be a lot of projection.

The first environmental physician I went to see listened to my story, sat back in her chair and said, "It's obvious that you don't want to get well." I was devastated. I later learned that she had cancer and her friends were angry with her because she put off getting help for it, so I believe she was projecting some of her issues onto me because I was also a physician. Later, we did have a more satisfying telephone conversation, after my blood tests showed that my thyroid was not functioning properly.

After some adjustment problems I was able to take a thyroid medication, in small amounts. That was a pivotal point, and I was able to expand the foods I could eat. By January 1990 I was up to six foods, including a grain, which I hadn't been able to eat in a year and a half. I worked up to being able to stand and walk for up to an hour a day. That period lasted about three months, until one day a nerve in my foot became so inflamed that when I stepped out of my car it felt like a tack was rammed into my foot. I've never really recovered from that relapse, which happened ten years ago.

In the meantime, I had gone to see an immunologist experienced in treating patients with MCS. He had a reputation for heroic acts and going to bat for people. I had to have somebody drive me there and somebody else carry me in, I was so sick and weak. He examined me and said, "You probably have cancer." That wasn't very reassuring. It turned out that he believed MCS was a precursor to cancer, and that he also was friends with the first doctor I saw and another female physician who both had cancer. I believe that he also was doing some projecting onto me.

That's when I began to see a chiropractor and to work with kinesiology. Eventually I began to make connections between exposures and the symptoms I would have. Like, I realized at some point that when I was breathing car exhaust I got a metallic taste in my mouth, and a weird feeling in my muscles. My throat felt like it was starting to close when I ate certain foods. I learned to use muscle testing to avoid the foods that caused my worst reactions. I was terribly afraid that I would die of starvation. So I upped my prayers, trusted my intuition and continued trying to improve my health.

I stayed outside on that mat for five months, then in my car for

another six weeks. After that I moved into a house where I was laying down on that same mat, on a desktop in the living room. That
worked for me until I started being tormented by skunks. Not just
one skunk—there were skunks all over the county. In mating season you could smell them from five at night until ten the next morning. That went on continually for nine months, and it was really
making me sick. A lot of people don't realize this, but skunk spray
is a neurotoxic chemical. I tell you, this was such a part of my life
that I feel obligated to share this information with others. I was so
desperate, and there was no place I could go. I didn't know what
to do.

At times my mother drove me through the whole county looking for clean air. Sometimes we'd drive almost the whole night. One
crazy night she came and got me and we drove to the Berkeley
marina and tried to sleep in the car. That didn't work out, so we
parked in a parking lot at a suburban shopping center around dawn.
Right after we got there a work crew came and started painting. I
put towels over my head, trying to protect myself from the fumes.
I thought: What in the hell am I going to do? I had to have a protective barrier. So, we went back to where I lived and started making
one. A friend came and helped me create a tent out of aluminum
foil, with two air filters inside. I crammed myself into that tent with
a phone and flashlight, and stayed there for sixteen hours every day.
I called it a "burrito bag."

Fortunately, I can focus to a fault—which helped me to survive
that experience. I focus on what I'm doing and don't think about
what I'd really rather be doing. I focused on what I could do, rather
than what I couldn't. Many times I would go through a meditation
of everything that was working in my body, even though I felt like
a total wreck. Instead of thinking, Oh my God, I've got stomach
pains and my head hurts! I'd think, Well, I can wriggle my left big
toe. Good. I can wriggle my other toes. Good. I was able to pee
today. Good.

By the time I went through this whole litany covering my entire
body, I thought I was doing pretty well. A real conscious effort to
focus on the positive, on what is working, is an important coping
tool. If you don't, you'll go absolutely crazy.

I did a lot of thinking and a lot of praying, and read a lot of
inspirational books through clear vegetable bags to minimize my
reactions to the books. As long as I could get out of that confinement

once a day to eat, I was okay. But one day the skunk smell never cleared. That day I finally snapped. I called my mother and asked her to come and get me, and she did. I lived in the car in my parents' driveway until I was strong enough to tolerate a bedroom inside. I stayed at my parents' house for eight months.

When I first went out in public after living in isolation for a couple of years, I was so thrilled to be out I couldn't have cared less if people looked at me strangely because I was wearing a respirator. All I could think was, I'm so excited! After a while, though, it became more of a challenge. Like one time at a farmers' market when a man came up to me, put his face right into mine and said, "Smile!" To me, that was so patronizing! I doubt that he would go up and say that to a person struggling to get through a crowd in a wheelchair.

Another time I encountered a group of teens on the street in Santa Barbara. After they crossed the street one of the girls turned around and yelled, "You've lost it, lady!" My attendant ran over and handed her a flyer explaining why I was wearing a respirator.

On the hopeful side, sometimes when children are staring at me and ask their mothers, "What is that?" I've heard mothers respond to them by saying matter-of-factly: "Some people react to certain things," like it was no big deal.

Then there was a kid who crouched down to watch me walking through a store with my respirator on, and called to his friend to take a look. They turned to each other and said in unison, "Cool!"

Weird looks aren't so bad. To me the most painful experiences have been with people who are patronizing. They act like they care and believe you when they really don't. One of the worst examples I can think of was an anesthesiologist at the hospital where I had to have eye surgery a while back. The hospital did an incredible job of accommodating me. They allowed me to register in advance, and to bring my own oxygen and IV tubing and my own IV fluid. It had been ten years since I had taken any medications other than thyroid medicine, and I had been known to have severe reactions to some. So of course I was terrified, having no idea what would happen. I asked the anesthesiologist to give me the lowest possible dose of the anesthetic, which he told me was preservative-free. Come to find out, he was just humoring me. The anesthetic wasn't preservative-free, and he gave me a linebacker's dose which knocked me out into a black hole. Fortunately I had no other adverse reactions, but I felt painfully violated. Then later, when I was profusely thanking the rest of the staff for their efforts to accommodate me, one guy said, "Yeah, well, the mind can play a lot of tricks on you." I thought: You mean they did this because they thought I was out of my mind? On the one hand I didn't care why they did it, I had to have it done. But still, it was a gut-wrenching, sickening, humiliating experience to find out some of them were just humoring me.

Knowing that I'm educating people gives me purpose and keeps me from dwelling on my own problems. My experiences with living with MCS keep me on the pulse of what is happening to others and reminds me of how important it is for me to continue my work as an MCS educator and advocate.

Most of my friends stopped communicating with me when I got so sick that summer. Some of them said it was just too difficult for them to handle, others just faded away. Although that was very painful, I understood. For a while I was pretty much alone with my core self and my higher power. I took that opportunity to strengthen my relationship with God. Work that I had done in a 12-step program had given me a spiritual framework that sustained me when this illness hit. I credit the 12-step principles for keeping me on the sane side through that period. I also developed a new support system of people with MCS.

My mother really came to my rescue, although at first she couldn't imagine what was wrong with me or why I didn't just get up. Once she began to understand, with the help of my sister, she was incredible. She drove an hour each way, three days a week, to take care of me. She also hired an attendant for me until I received county in-home care services.

I was seeing a therapist who was helpful to me during that time. I think she was bewildered and horrified by what was happening to me, but she accepted it and respected my medical judgment that I was sick. We usually talked on the phone or, a few times, she came to visit me and we talked in the yard or in my car.

I had been in the habit of networking by phone, so I used that skill to network with other people who were environmentally ill. I became friends with Randa, who was then living in San Francisco and was active in the MCS community.

Randa and I moved to Santa Barbara together in '92. I had a lot of friends there and I was thrilled to be back, but some of my friends weren't as sensitive to my condition as I would have liked.

One of my friends invited Randa and me to attend her wedding rehearsal, but she wouldn't refrain from wearing perfume or ask the other guests to refrain, even though there were only a few people. We couldn't go into the church because the perfume was so horrendous, so we stood on the planter boxes with our noses pressed against the windows, watching from outside. Part of me was happy just to be able to watch, and part of me was hurt because she wasn't willing to accommodate us.

Even my best friend from my medical training, now an internist and head of a hospital department, still doesn't understand. He cares about me, but he'll say, "Don't you think you could just expose yourself a little more at a time to get desensitized?" I tell him to drop dead, and I've given him information on MCS and related articles I've written.

While Randa and I lived in a one-room guest house on the outskirts of Santa Barbara, my health continued to improve until the day a maintenance guy dumped Dursban in our yard. They were having trouble with flies in the main house, so he'd made an extra-strong batch of Dursban and sprayed it in the house. He was told it was too strong and to get rid of it. That's when he tossed it in our backyard. It was summertime and our windows were open. Both Randa and I are extremely sensitive to pesticides. When those fumes drifted in we took one breath, ran from the house, jumped in the car and left. A friend—who didn't have MCS and happened to be visiting at the time—dug up the contaminated dirt and disposed of it further away from our house. When we went back everything in the house was contaminated. So we set up a hotplate in the driveway, Randa pitched a tent and I slept in the car. We carried as much as we could outside to bake in the sun, and the house was scrubbed with TSP [trisodium phosphate]. We found that we could touch some of our papers and things without our fingers burning from the pesticide residue after they sat out in the sun for five or six days. But we finally gave up and decided to try living someplace else, because Randa wasn't doing well there anyway because of the pollen and mold.

We wanted to check out towns in Arizona and New Mexico. I was too sick to drive, so my attendant drove us in her father's RV. We looked at several areas, and when we found a sublet in Santa Fe we went home, packed our things and moved.

It didn't take long for us to learn that housing problems would continue to be a challenge here. One house we rented had a bad roof that had to be re-tarred. After that it was ten months before I could sleep in the house. We tried to make it safe with foil barriers on the ceiling, but it just didn't work. We kept the windows open—even in the winter—so I could be in the house during the day. But I went to a friend's house every night to sleep on the floor through the winter, then slept in my car for another five months when the weather was better.

Sometimes I call these kinds of experiences "lab work." They are a constant reminder of what it's like to live with MCS and why it's so important to educate others about this disease.

In order to deal with the tragedy of this illness in my life, I've embraced the idea that things happen for a reason. People with MCS have been shown something that other people can only imagine. Knowing a chemical can cause cancer in twenty-five years is pretty nebulous. We breathe the same chemical and we're knocked on our asses. We've crossed an invisible line, and our lives are not the same.

I believe my life was spared for a purpose, and that purpose is to use my knowledge and my skills to bring awareness to this issue. In June of '96 I was asked by the New Mexico Governor's Committee on Concerns for the Handicapped to organize a "Town Hall" meeting on MCS in Santa Fe. We had twenty panelists from state agencies and a hundred and twenty people in the audience, most of whom were chemically sensitive. We went to great pains to make it as accessible as possible. We had a fragrance sniffer at the door, phone-in access for people who couldn't attend, a microphone and speaker outside on the patio for those who had to stay outside the building, and organic food for lunch. The speakers addressed pesticides, housing, health care, employment and school issues. After each speaker we took comments from the audience, so we heard from fifty or sixty chemically-sensitive people. It packed quite a punch. That really was a catalyst for launching our advocacy work here.

As a result of that we got involved with the state's Department of Education to produce an MCS awareness brochure that went out to all the school administrators. That work led to invitations to four pesticide conferences, and to the opportunity to work on drafting regulations for pesticide notification. We also got involved with the Department of Health and participated in an MCS prevalence study working group. One of the outcomes of that was the inclusion of questions regarding chemical sensitivity on a statewide survey. That study revealed that sixteen percent of the population in New Mexico consider themselves unusually sensitive to common everyday chemicals, two percent have been diagnosed with MCS, and two percent have lost a job or career because of chemical sensitivities. These statistics show that MCS is a widespread public health problem.

I'm particularly interested in educating the medical profession. It is very hard for some doctors to accept that there are people who vomit blood, or have a convulsion, or a cardiovascular reaction to low levels of pesticide exposure. It's terribly disturbing to have people in positions of influence say there is nothing wrong with us, when that is so far from the truth. Last year the editor of a medical journal rejected information on the prevalence of MCS in Gulf War veterans because he didn't believe the illness existed. It's like saying the Holocaust didn't happen.

Sometimes when I read or hear about these incidents it's so disheartening that my first thought is: This is so depressing that I can't even respond to it. But I know how this biased information filters down to affect people with MCS in their daily lives, and how it is being used against us in the courts. Since I write and speak well, I've been quite successful in getting my views published, so I feel duty-bound to give it my best effort. Pretty soon after reading something that is terribly depressing I start to think: Maybe I can at least make this point, or, I could get so-and-so to write a letter, or I'll send copies to folks so they'll see what we're up against.

I'm told that I have a personality that enables me to relate to a lot of different kinds of people. People seem to think of me as a good ambassador. In a strange way I'm easygoing with a very intense core, and I'm passionate about the polluted state of the world. When I get riled by anti–MCS articles, I usually get it out by writing critical letters to the editor.

Doctors are so busy worrying that they might be fooled into thinking people with MCS are really sick when they're not, that they don't realize they've been fooled by a disinformation campaign by the pharmaceutical companies. Doctors pride themselves on being independent of the pharmaceutical industry, on not being influenced by them in any way. The day that they understand how badly they've been duped they're going to jump to our side. Like me, most doctors are shocked to learned how many pharmaceutical companies make pesticides, and to what extent they are controlling the information that doctors receive.

More doctors are taking an interest in this illness. That gives me hope. Here in New Mexico we got signatures from forty doctors in two weeks to support legislation to fund an MCS awareness program.

One message we try to stress in our awareness campaign is that people with MCS are like everybody else. Most of us were average, healthy folks. This illness is found in every age group, every race, every ethnicity, and every socioeconomic class. Everybody is at risk. We are trying to prevent others from getting sick.

Through our efforts here in Santa Fe, the city council voted unanimously to adopt an Integrated Pest Management program and phase out the city's use of pesticides. The council applauded us for our contribution to the community with this work. I think it was clear to the policymakers and community that we were not just working for ourselves. I want people to understand that—that the MCS advocacy community is not just advocating for people with the illness—we're working to prevent children and adults from getting MCS and other toxic injuries. It was so moving to me to be recognized by the city council for making a difference in the community, to go from living in a foil-lined tent to making a contribution to the community. I am very grateful for having been given this opportunity.

Most of my time is spent in my bedroom reading, writing and talking on the phone. I still can eat only nine foods. I have to be very careful about what I eat and breathe. I have to stay away from people who are ill because a virus could stop me from eating. I come into town about twice a week and can go into one health food store. I hardly go anyplace else. I actually have more restrictions now, in terms of places I can go, than I used to. Two years ago I started having heart problems after I went into the capitol building to testify, so I won't go back there. Occasionally I used to go into a smoke-free bar or coffeehouse—wearing a respirator—to listen to music, but I haven't been able to do that in a while. A couple of times I played the drums in a women's jazz trio. That was when I still couldn't sit because of my back, so I played standing up and could only tap lightly, but I could keep the beat. Those were big outings for me.

It's always a real possibility that I will die from this illness. There have been times when I wasn't sure I would make it. Like when I developed an eye infection. My face swelled up with cellulitis, and I knew full well that it could kill me if I didn't start taking an antibiotic. I also knew, from previous reactions to medications, that there was a real chance the antibiotic could kill me. I called the local hospital and told the hospital personnel that I was going to take the antibiotic sitting in my car in the hospital's parking lot in case anything happened to me. They said, "We won't come out to see you, you'll have to have somebody carry you in if you have a problem." So three friends went with me, and I prayed a lot. I did okay on the antibiotic for a while, then had a reaction but it wasn't life-threatening.

Coming to grips with death was a turning point for me. During my first year of having MCS, when my fear of death was so intense, I made peace with the idea that I might not live. It has given me more freedom to take risks when necessary, but not unreasonable risks.

One of the reasons I work so hard on advocacy is that I know that my mental clarity, the food I can eat, and the safety of my home could all be taken away in a second. I don't want to look back and think, I was watching television when I could have called somebody from the Department of Health and might have made a difference.

When I get calls from people who are terrified and desperate, I tell them that most of us with MCS have gone through incredibly horrible situations where it looked like there was no way out. But people make their way out. All you can do is have faith in God— or some higher power—believe there is a plan for you, try to stay open and follow the path the best that you can. I tell people that I believe in the ultimate good of the universe, and that no matter how far down the scale you go, you can always use your experience to help others.

I encourage people to look at this as a disability rather than a medical crisis they can fix. Susan Molloy and other Bay Area disability advocates introduced me to the disability model of coping, with a focus on the here and now, accepting the capabilities that you have and doing the best you can with them. This is much more productive, I believe, than waiting until you find a "cure" to live your life again.

Why would anyone expect to recover completely when very few people do? One of the most poignant quotes I've heard was "One guy told me he has completely recovered from MCS—twice." It's more productive to think about this illness as being more like diabetes than the flu. If your doctor and your family members think you can just get over this, they're going to be mad at you when you don't. People with other disabilities—like those who are paraplegic or blind—generally don't put their lives on hold waiting for a cure. They look at what they can do and get on with life. You have to start with where you are and go from there.

It really helps the process a lot if I have a sense of humor, if I can laugh at how unbelievably bizarre my life can be with MCS. I've had to have my attendants wrap their heads in hats and plastic bags when the chemicals in their hair products made me ill. I knew one woman who asked her mother to wrap her head in aluminum foil. Then there was the time when a television news crew came to interview me, as a physician, for a feature on environmental illness. There I was, flat on my back in the backseat of my car with a camera in my face. I spoke in a calm, professional manner, as though it was perfectly normal to be living horizontally in my car. When that seems normal, you know you've stepped over to the other side!

A friend of mine asks, "Do you really expect people to understand this illness?" We call it the Total Creative Lifestyle, because, with MCS, you can't do anything the way you used to. You can't clean your clothes the same way. You can't shop the same. You can't hang out with the same people. This is actually very traumatic, but if you embrace the creative part of it, it's much more positive.

Another name we have for MCS is the Wasted Money Disease, because we spend so much money on things that don't work out, like housing, food, clothing, medications, cars, beds, computers— you name it.

In closing I'd just like to say, Keep the faith!

Erica Elliott
Santa Fe, New Mexico

Board certified in family practice and environmental medicine, Erica Elliott, M.D., has a private practice and lives in an adobe-style cohousing community surrounded by cacti, footpaths, and creative energy on the edge of Santa Fe.

An active and robust child from a heritage of Swiss physicians, Erica was raised on whole foods and a wholesome lifestyle. Her father's career as an army general led her family to live in many locations. She began school in England, graduated from high school in Germany, and attended college in the U.S. She speaks eight languages.

Before entering medical school Erica taught bilingual education on the Navajo Indian reservation, then worked and lived as a sheepherder. She served in the Peace Corps in Ecuador and was the first American woman to reach the summit of Mt. Aconcagua in Argentina, the highest mountain in the western hemisphere. She also led various groups on wilderness expeditions and taught Outward Bound for three summers. She led an all women's expedition to the top of Mt. McKinley in 1980 and had a peak named after her in Ecuador after she did a first ascent of the peak.

At age thirty-one Erica began medical school at the University of Colorado. She completed a three-year family practice residency in a Denver hospital, then went to Cuba, New Mexico, where she served as the medical director of a rural hospital as repayment for her National Health Service scholarship. After serving in that capacity she was married for two years. She has one son who is now ten years old.

The rural hospital where I worked had only nine beds, a very busy emergency room and outpatient clinic. We were treating Navajos, Hispanic ranchers and Anglos. It was an incredible experience. Night after night I stayed up delivering babies. It was exhausting and I was so incredibly sleep deprived that there were times when I would actually be asleep with my eyes open. I was working these long hours and trying to raise my son. By this time he was calling the baby-sitter "Mommy" and that was heartbreaking to me. So I decided to go to work for an HMO in Santa Fe, a multi-specialty clinic in a new building. This was before I knew anything about sick building syndrome and chemical sensitivity.

I thought my life would be easier because I was only working fifty hours a week, as opposed to eighty or a hundred. I was on night duty only one night a week—which was a huge improvement—and I had more time with my son. But after I started working there in

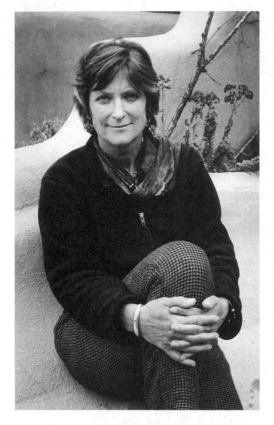

January of '91, I felt exhausted. I thought I must really hate my job because I felt like I would pass out at work, but on the weekends I was fine.

I had always counted on my excellent health and resiliency, and had enormous endurance and reserves from my days as a mountain climber. And, my background is Swiss, so in my family you just try harder and harder. In spite of that my health kept going downhill. I reached a point where I had no reserves. I was out of steam. Yet, I kept denying it until I felt sick all the time—not just at work—and it started to affect my brain and nervous system. I felt so confused all the time. Sometimes when I was driving I didn't even know what city I was in or where I lived, because of the fumes—but I didn't know that was the reason at the time. I'd pull over to the side of the road and slap myself and say, "Come on! Snap out of it! You know where you are!"

Every time I tried to figure out what was wrong, I was at a complete loss. I went to see different physicians, who all thought I must be depressed. I was put on Prozac and my health continued to worsen. I was sinking fast.

My brain was so far gone at that point, I couldn't track a conversation or hold a thought. My short-term memory was gone. I was relying on my nurse to cover for me. She wasn't as sick as I was, because I was exposed to fumes in the treatment room *and* in my office.

Several events happened that helped me to start putting the pieces together, to figure out that I had multiple chemical sensitivity. I really don't remember the exact sequence of events, because I was in such a fog at the time.

One turning point for me was when a new doctor came to town from Hawaii. He sent a letter to all the physicians in the community about his practice in environmental medicine and the kinds of patients he saw. I had never heard of it, but his letter caught my attention. The patients he described sounded like me. I was still in the closet about my condition because I was so frightened about what was happening to me. So I called him up and said, "I have some patients like this and I'd like to understand this better. Can we have lunch together?" At lunch I finally confessed. In tears I said, "This is happening to me. Can you help me?" He said, "Yes," and he started educating me. That's when I thought maybe I would live.

There also was a Medicare patient I saw, completely disabled by MCS, who helped to educate me. He was rambling on about his problems when all of a sudden he stopped and very compassionately said, "Dr. Elliott, what is wrong with you?" He said it in such a way that I was defenseless and started to cry. I cried and cried and cried. He put his arm around me and said, "Tell me about it." All the fears I'd been holding in came spilling out to this person whom I didn't even know. I couldn't pretend anymore. My whole body heaved as two years of holding back let go into this endless flood of sobbing. I said, "I'm dying." And I reeled off all these symptoms I was having. He said, "You've got sick building syndrome. Do you know what that is?" I said, "Not really." He said, "The building is making you sick." I said, "I know." He said, "Why are you still here?" I sobbed, "Because if I quit I won't be able to feed my son, and if I can't take care of my son I might as well kill myself." My brain was so far gone I couldn't problem solve. I did this black and white thinking—either I stayed in the job or I'd live in the streets.

"Okay, we have to get a plan," he said. "First, you have to read this book by Sherry Rogers called *Tired or Toxic?*"

I said, "I can't read. I can't even hold a thought."

"Okay, just hold it then. Keep it by your bed and just look at it, even if you don't remember a thing. Once in a while just open it up before you go to sleep and it will give you comfort." Then he said, "We need to get you out of this building. I want you to resign immediately." I said, "I can't do that!" He said, "You *have* to. Look, I'm going to make an appointment to come back in two weeks, to check on you." In two weeks he came back and said, "What is your plan?" I said, "I don't know." He said, "If you don't leave I'm going to the newspaper to report what is going on in this building."

I got so angry. I said, "You betrayed me! If you do that, I'm going to get fired!" He said, "That's the point. If you're not going to go on your own, I'm going to do whatever it takes to get you out of this building." I said, "Okay, okay, just give me a little more time!"

It was also during that period that I began to notice that other people in the building were complaining of burning eyes and throat, and other problems. One day I saw my nurse staggering out of the procedure room with tears streaming down her face. Her face was bright red, but she wasn't crying. I said, "Michelle, what's wrong?" She said, "Oh, I'm always like this when I come out of the procedure room." I said, "What is it?" And she said, "Chemicals." That's when I really started to pay attention to what was in the building.

I noticed that once a month I felt like I had the flu, which turned out I learned later to coincide with monthly applications of pesticides in the building. I also noticed a putrid smell, periodically, from the ceiling. I called the manager but the smell was gone when she finally came several hours later. She thought I had imagined it.

I think the fact that I was so doggedly determined—which got me to the top of mountains and through medical school—kept me from doing what I should have done right away, which was to say: Even though I don't know what's wrong, I need to get out of this building.

Finally I insisted that they call someone to do an inspection. A building inspector came and didn't find anything wrong, so I kept insisting they call him back. When he came back again I said, "I know there's something wrong with this building! We're all sick. You've got to find it!"

He found that the gluteraldehyde levels from the disinfectant we used were way too high, the formaldehyde levels in the building were too high, and the ventilation was faulty. He discovered that the exhaust for the HVAC system was located on the roof right next to the intake, so every time the wind blew from the west it funneled the fumes right back into the building. Because of where my office was located, I got hit the hardest.

Never will I forget the day I finally resigned. A patient came in wearing perfume that day. She sat on the exam table, talking on and on. I couldn't even focus my eyes. I was seeing double. I was so embarrassed about my condition because I didn't know what was wrong with me, and I didn't want anyone to know how seriously damaged I was because I didn't have a plan for how I could manage without my job. When she finished talking she asked me, "What should I do?" I had no idea what she had been talking about. My face was flushed, my heart was racing and my eyes were burning. It was a nightmare. I said, "My nurse will follow up with you."

After she walked out, I picked up the phone, called the director and said, "I have to resign. I can't go on. I'm afraid I'm going to make a mistake and harm somebody." He said, "What do you mean?" I said, "I'm so sick I think I am dying." He said, "What's wrong with you?" I said, "I've told you many times." Every time I'd told him something was wrong with me he had said, "Oh, you just have the flu." I had said, "No, I don't have the flu. Nobody has the flu non-stop. It doesn't go away anymore. I'm sick all the time." Now he said, "You just need a vacation." I said, "I can't stay. I'm going to make a terrible mistake and injure somebody." I quit on June 1, 1993.

The next few years were a gradual climb out of that hell. I used to cry every night, and took comfort in the thought that I could die if I wanted to. I would never commit suicide, but just knowing that was an option was comforting. That's not even in my thoughts today. I'm not the same woman I was when my body crashed between '91 and '93.

When I first left that job I thought I'd have to go on welfare. I thought I was useless. Then the medical director of a women's health clinic called and asked me to work for her. She told me they would be willing to accommodate me by asking patients to refrain from wearing fragrances, putting air filters in my room and allowing me to keep the windows open and to heat my office with an electric space heater. She said they would instruct the maintenance crew to clean only with vinegar and water, and they would request that no pesticides or herbicides be used in or near the building. And she said I could work part time, with no night hours, and no hospital duty—the hospital was too toxic for me. I was amazed and grateful. It came just in the nick of time to keep me from losing my house.

Working there was terribly hard because I was still so sick, and patients came in wearing fragrances despite their efforts. Still, I could limp by, even though I was miserable. But the practice grew and we needed a larger space. I knew that if we moved into a new building that would be a deathblow for me, so I started to see a few MCS patients in my home in case the new building didn't work out. When a larger space was located, I was told it would have to be remodeled.

They agreed to use any nontoxic materials I wanted, but some toxic products were used accidentally. I lasted one hour after we moved into the building, I was so sick. Since then I have been seeing patients only in my home.

I was always a closet alternative practitioner. Now everyone in town knows that's my forte. People who come to me want alternatives to conventional medications. They want a different approach. Many come just to ask me to share with them what I've done to help myself. What I tell them, and what I tell myself, is that there is a bigger picture here. We are not alone in our suffering. The wildlife is getting sick or becoming extinct and the soils are depleted. This is about all of us. It's not personal. There's something I find comforting in that thought.

I tell them about how I was lost to the bigger picture, how I wanted to die, and how grateful I am now to be alive, because I have something valuable to offer that would have been lost if I had killed myself. Patients tell me that my story has inspired them to not give up.

After I had partially recovered I got board certified in environmental medicine. Now I'm certified in both family practice and environmental medicine. I think most people are affected by chemicals. Those of us with MCS are just on one end of the spectrum. I see patients with MS, rheumatoid arthritis, fibromyalgia and other conditions, and there's almost always a chemical link someplace in their complaints. I always keep an eye out for that aspect contributing to these illnesses.

Being self-employed is sometimes terrifying. Like this winter, when I got really sick with an infection and it went on and on through November, December, January and February. My practice really dwindled and I couldn't pay my bills. The terror makes me more ill, because strong emotions are toxic to me.

I have a friend who is really helpful to me when I get into fearful thinking like that. I talk to her about the cognitive part. It also helps me to meditate and to exercise. It's hard for me to hold onto worry when I'm exercising. If I have the energy to exercise it's a wonderful antidote to that gripping fear.

I'm so happy now that I can practice the kind of medicine that I believe in. By practicing in my home I have more control over my environment and my schedule, and I have more time with my son. If I had never gotten sick I might still be working at an HMO because of the reasonable pay, good hours and benefits, and because of the dogma in the medical community that prevents doctors from moving away from conventional medicine. They're so afraid that if they get off this track they'll be rejected and despised by their colleagues. But that's starting to shift. Alternative medicine is getting more acceptance.

When I fell off the treadmill I felt like a leper with no worth. I lost a lot of friends because I wasn't the same Erica they had known. Now some of my old friends are coming back, and that's all right.

In the old days I felt so rejected and abandoned when my needs weren't understood. Now I have a different view, a much broader perspective. I'm more forgiving when people don't understand, or when they think I'm crazy, or too demanding, or irritable, or paranoid, because this illness is so strange that it is beyond their realm of comprehension. I could be in their shoes. In fact, before I got ill I was ignorant about these things, too.

In retrospect I realize that I was seeing chemically sensitive patients for years, but I was too ignorant to recognize what I was seeing. Neither I nor they knew what was wrong. Like many doctors, I was treating symptoms and not getting at the problem at all. I was bound by time constraints. I saw up to sixty patients a day, which allowed me approximately ten minutes for each patient. With that kind of schedule all you're doing is throwing medications at different symptoms. I feel I did nothing to help those people, and might have made them worse. The only thing I offered that was different from other doctors was that I listened. I would take them seriously and not immediately refer them to a psychiatrist.

When I was first injured not many doctors had ever heard of this illness. Those who knew me before I was injured believed me because they knew me and knew my credibility. Now my colleagues are inviting me to speak on multiple chemical sensitivity. I spoke to a group of one hundred doctors at the hospital. I was so sick that I had to read the entire presentation, but it was well received. Since then I have received many invitations to speak to health care professionals all over. Now when I ask a roomful of doctors how many have heard of MCS, everyone in the room raises their hand.

The most difficult losses for me have been the things I took the most pride in, like my athletic ability. Mountain climbing was my passion. I was a world-class athlete, and I lost my coordination. I also used to take so much pride in my brain. I knew what people were going to say even before they said it. I lost that when I was injured, and had to start practicing more from my heart. I think that is what one patient was talking about when she told me "I like you better since you've been sick." Another patient, the one who told me I had to leave the HMO, later wrote to me and said, "Of all the doctors I've seen, you helped me the most because you were so real with me." I think patients are hungry for that.

This house I'm living in has had a lot to do with my recovery. I had started building this just before I left my job at the HMO. It was terrifying to feel like I could no longer work, when this house was under construction. My life was so uncertain, especially financially. Somehow, though, I managed. And, fortunately, I learned enough about environmental illness in time to make wise choices in terms of building products. It also helped that the architect is somewhat chemically sensitive, so the cohousing community was designed to be more environmentally friendly than most places. My brain was so impaired that half the time I had no idea what the architect was talking about. I tried to compensate for my deficits by being a sweet, compliant person. I would just smile and agree with what she said, because you have to know what's going on in order to raise any questions.

When I moved in I posted signs everywhere in the community asking people to refrain from using fabric softeners and scented detergents, and explaining my illness. Although not everyone honors my request, most of the people have gotten used to being fragrance-free and no longer like the scented products. A couple of nights a week we have community dinners, and it was a struggle, at first, to get everyone to agree to make them organic.

My goals now are to be the best mother I can be for my son, to continue to offer help and comfort to patients, to develop my spiritual life, and to increase awareness of environmental health issues. We've made a lot of progress in raising awareness in Santa Fe. It's been a group effort spearheaded by Ann McCampbell. We started with the schools. After months and months of hounding public school administrators, they agreed to stop the monthly spraying of pesticides, but only when they realized it would save them thousands of dollars if they used chemicals only as needed. From there, Ann started working on getting pesticides out of the parks. Pretty soon she was talking to all the city council members and to the governor. Since then the city has adopted an Integrated Pest Management (IPM) program and has begun phasing out the use of pesticides in public buildings, and they have created an IPM Coordinator position. Recently, at one of their public meetings the city council acknowledged Ann for her efforts to protect people from the harmful effects of chemicals. Our next project is to focus on hospitals. We've already made lots of inroads. We've planted seeds, talked to all of the ICU nurses, the home health nurses and others.

I'm hoping our progress in Santa Fe will inspire others to not feel helpless, and to make changes in other communities.

We are using our illness as a way to enhance our lives by offering something important to the world. We can all use this nightmare as a way to serve others.

Tomasita Gallegos Santa Fe, New Mexico

Born and raised in Santa Fe, Tomasita Gallegos has lived and worked in the same community all her life. Work was a source of great pride to her and she always enjoyed good health, until she was exposed to an unidentified toxin in her workplace at age thirty-three. Now she relies on her faith in God, her family, the compassion of her former employer, and disability income to survive. She rarely leaves her house.

Like many people with MCS, Tomasita's emotions are affected by chemical exposures. Still recovering from a recent exposure when I interviewed her, she was feeling emotionally fragile but welcomed me into her home on short notice. In a soft voice she told to me her story, unable at times to hold back her tears.

Without the compassionate, ethical support of her former employer, Tomasita's life would be dramatically different. Sadly, for every person like Tomasita there are many more whose employers deny the reality of MCS, leaving disabled workers without a source of income for adequate food, housing or medical care.

Tomasita is a gentle and sincere woman with two children, a teenaged daughter and a married son. And she is thrilled to now be a grandmother.

I've always worked. I worked in a nursing home as a nurses' aide, then I went into private duty taking care of elderly people in their homes. I was healthy. I went out in public and people came into my home and I didn't have to worry about what anybody was wearing. I had a pretty good life. Then everything changed.

I had been working for the same woman for three years when I had an exposure at work that made me ill. To this day we're not really sure what it was, even though my employer has had all kinds of scientists come to do testing to try to figure out what happened to me. She and my brother also have been affected by whatever it was. In my heart I believe a guest who stayed there used a pesticide in the guest house and threw the container in the trash compactor. I had gone into that guest house daily with no problems until this day in February of 1993.

My employer was very strict about what was brought into her house. She suffered with chronic fatigue, so she didn't allow us to wear perfume or fabric softener on our clothes and didn't allow us to come to work if we were ill. The day after the guest left I wasn't at work. When I came back the following day my brother, who also worked for her—and still does—told me he had smelled perfume in the guest house. We figured the guest had used something even though everyone knew it made this woman sick. When I went into the guest house to get a magazine for my employer, I smelled the perfume. I didn't think much about it because the smell of perfume had never bothered me. In fact, I wore perfume on my days off work. I picked up the magazine and left, and went back to my employer's house. Later, at twenty minutes to five, I decided to go back and mop the kitchen floor in the guest house because I had twenty more minutes to work. While I was filling a bucket with water the smell of perfume became more and more intense and my skin started burning, but I still didn't pay any attention. While I was mopping I kept brushing my hair back from my face, and accidentally I hit the trash compactor. Then the smell became even more intense, the muscles in my neck tied up in knots and I could taste the perfume in my mouth. It was a horrible perfume taste and I started to salivate like a bulldog and became extremely paranoid. I rushed to finish mopping. Then I went back to my employer's house and told her what had happened. I was crying and feeling very emotional and afraid. My face felt like it was drooping, like a dentist had given me a shot. I didn't know what was going on and I was so scared. My employer told me to go on home. When I got in my car and started driving I was so scared and I was crying. I kept salivating, and I didn't know if I was driving in the right direction. I had to pull my car off the road for a while. Finally I got home and started pulling off my

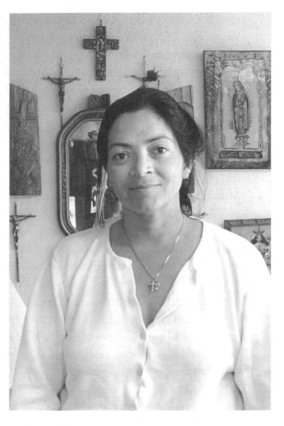

clothes on the way into the house. My husband and kids wanted to know what was wrong. I told them I didn't know and explained what had happened, then I took a shower—which helped a little—and went to bed and cried myself to sleep.

The next day I still didn't feel well but I went back to work. My joints and body ached all over and my face and skin were blotchy. No one was allowed to go into the guest house. When I went into the laundry room I felt worse, but I didn't understand I was reacting to the laundry products. I also felt worse when I folded the laundry. I thought maybe I was coming down with a cold because it was winter and many people were sick. That night I went home and spent the evening in bed.

The day after that I went back to work and went into the guest house to empty the trash compactor. The smell wasn't gone but it didn't seem as strong as it had before. Then, when I got the trash, I had the same reaction as before. My face felt numb, my muscles tensed, my skin burned, I salivated and I felt extremely paranoid and emotional. I went back to my employer's house crying, and she saw right away that something was wrong again.

This went on and on with me getting sick at work and at home, and I was like a crazy person. When I tried to cook on my gas stove I'd see spiders crawling all over the place. We had to disconnect it and I cooked on a hotplate. I was hearing voices and seeing things. My whole body itched and felt like insects were crawling all over me. Eventually I learned it was my nervous system making me feel that way, but I didn't know it then. I actually thought there were millions of flies on me.

My kids were afraid of me. They'd sit by me and I'd get sick. My son was a teenager then, so he was wearing cologne. My kids would bring me a glass of water and I thought they were trying to poison me because the water made me sick. Or they would sit next to me and I got sick because they were wearing products I reacted to, but I didn't understand that.

In March I asked to take some time off work to clean my house, because I thought I had brought something from there that had contaminated my house. I cleaned my whole house—the walls, woodwork and everything—with an industrial strength disinfectant. That only made me worse.

I went to see my doctor five times and to urgent care. None of them knew what was wrong. They basically told me it was all in my head because I was in a bad marriage. My daughter, who was eight at the time, wrote me a note telling me she was sorry I had gone crazy.

Finally, my employer sent me to an allergist who told me I had had some kind of a chemical exposure, and he told me what to wear to go back in there to clean it up. He told me to wear all cotton, long sleeves and a mask. But I didn't go back to the guest house or back to work.

I felt like a magnet, like everything was coming off from other people onto me. I became suicidal and wanted to die. I took a bunch of pills and had to have my stomach pumped. I thought there was no help and no hope. That's when my family physician told me that he thought Dr. Erica Elliott could help me. My husband and brother went with me to see her. She told us she had an illness caused by exposure to chemicals, and that the same thing had happened to me. I was so relieved I cried. I was so happy to find out I wasn't crazy.

Dr. Elliott was so sick herself at that time that she sent me to someone else for treatment. But she told us I couldn't go back home, and that I should not drink the city water because I would react to chemicals in the water.

I lived in a tent in my brother's backyard for a month, until I started reacting to the materials he was using to build a house. Then I lived in a hotel for another month. My family went in first to strip the sheets and everything. I slept in a sleeping bag.

I started reading and educating myself. We threw everything out of my house and my brother and family washed the whole house down with plain water, because I was even reacting to baking soda. Some of my things I brought back into the house after baking them off out in the sun. It's been a gradual thing to get my house back.

It was a complete change. My kids had to change, too. My son was a teenager and he had to stop wearing cologne. And he worked as a tiler so he had to take his clothes off outside and come in and take a shower as soon as he got home. It was hard for them and they resented it at first, but they could see how much better I did when I wasn't around chemicals.

My marriage didn't survive. My illness just added to the problems we already had, and my husband just didn't understand. I think he would have put me away if he could. For a long time I believed that if you loved someone and stuck it out that it would change. Finally I realized that I needed to get out of the marriage to take care of myself.

When I brushed my teeth my gums would swell and bleed, and I became allergic to a lot of foods that had never bothered me before. My diet changed dramatically. Yeast, dairy and wheat products make me sick. I had to start reading labels and shopping in the health food stores.

My former employer has been an angel. I don't know what I would do without her. She has helped me tremendously and still does. She paid my wages for a whole year and helped me to make my house payments after my husband moved out. I have to make sure I can make my house payments. I can't afford to lose my house because I can't live anywhere else. After three years of fighting I finally got disability income, which is basically just enough to make my house payments.

I filed for worker's compensation because my employer had paid for that. It took two years to get a hearing and the judge told me it was all in my head and that I was trying to get rich and he wasn't going to help me. So that ended there.

Not being able to support myself has been the biggest loss for me. I wish I could provide more for my daughter. She goes without a lot because I don't have the income. I've tried working and tried to think of work I can do in my home. I tried baby-sitting, but I couldn't stand the soaps and detergents on the children's skin and clothes. People feel offended when you tell them that sort of thing. I tried cleaning homes for other people with MCS, but I had to quit because what works for one person makes another person sick. One lady had a cat, and since my original exposure I've been terribly sensitive to cats and dogs. The lady said the cat didn't come into the part of the house where I was cleaning, but she didn't understand that she carried the cat's hair and dander from one part of the house to the other. I just couldn't do it anymore. I've tried working in different places but people come in wearing scents or I react to the buildings themselves. Even when I go to my family member's homes I have to leave after a few minutes. I have trouble going into anyone's house.

I would love to be able to go back to work for the same lady I worked for before. But she's a smoker and now I can't stand the smoke. My worst fear is that I will lose my house. I don't know what I'd do if I lost my home.

My brother has been my Rock of Gibraltar through all of this. He told me I wasn't crazy. I don't know what I would have done without him. He told me that he has been sensitive to perfume and other chemicals ever since he was exposed to Agent Orange when he was a marine in Vietnam. He said he never told us before because we wouldn't have believed him. I knew he was a different person since he came back from the war. He wouldn't let us use nail polish or hair spray and things like that when he was around us, and he wouldn't go to family functions unless they were outdoors. After he came back from Vietnam he didn't live with us for long. I was younger then and I just thought he was grouchy. After he was exposed to whatever it was in the guest house his reactions to other exposures became more intense and now it takes him longer to recover. He has learned to live with having reactions everywhere he goes.

His seven-year-old daughter, Juanita, is sensitive to chemicals, too. They had to pull the carpet out of her room because the foam padding was making her sick, and she reacts to perfumes and things like that. She goes through crying fits like I do. It's sad. At a family party Juanita came up to me and said, "Do you have MCS too?" I said yes, and she said, "So do I. It's good to know somebody else that has it, too." I just wanted to cry, because I know that feeling. It's sad that this is happening to people, and it's scary too, because people don't believe you. But it's not in our head. We're not making these things up.

None of the people I knew before I got sick have anything to do with me now. Either they don't understand or they don't believe me. They were friends with my ex-husband, too, so I'm sure he told them it was all in my head. I've come to accept the fact that if they were true friends they would try to help me.

I used to try to defend myself when people didn't believe me. I tried to explain what was happening to me. Now I just tell myself they are ignorant or in denial because they don't want to face the truth. But it hurts. I do have feelings, and it's not easy living with this disease. It's not easy at all.

My family and my boyfriend are my only friends now. When I met my boyfriend he was willing to change his lifestyle to accommodate me. I know he has a hard time because my emotions are so unpredictable. One minute I'm happy, one minute I'm sad. One minute I'm mad and ready to kill somebody. I can't help it. I open the door and I get sick.

That's why I'm telling you my story. I want more people to know about this, to be educated about MCS. I want them to know that things they wear can make other people sick. I also want people to know they can't get this disease from me, it's not contagious.

I try to help other people when I can. There's a lady who calls me because she built a new house and she got sick as soon as she moved in. One of my brothers was her plumber, and he told her to call me because he thought I could help. She's living in a storage room now.

I tell people not to give up. There is help out there. A lot of it has to do with changing your lifestyle, figuring out what you react to and avoiding those things. We all react to different things.

I tell people it's not in their head, there are things in the environment that are making them sick. I tell them how it has helped me to change all the products I use and to avoid exposures to chemicals. If I go into a store or someplace else and it smells bad, I leave. I used to be very afraid to do that because people would say, "What's bothering you? There's nothing bothering me." Like my aunt. I love her to pieces but she's an elderly lady and she can't understand why I can't stand her soaps.

I try to shop early in the morning or late in the evening when there aren't as many people in the stores. But even then it is hard. The other day I was standing in line and a lady got in line right behind me and was practically standing on top of me. I wanted to turn around and tell her to please move, because her hair spray was killing me. It felt like an hour before I could finish my business and leave. When you're reacting it feels like everything is dragging on. It really wasn't taking long, it just seemed that way because I was reacting. When I moved, she moved right with me.

I don't participate in school functions much now because I get terribly sick in schools. Once in a while I go out to dinner, during off-hours, and sit away from smoking areas and other people. I know what I can eat now and what I can't.

Working in my yard is good therapy for me. But I stay in the house a lot because we live so close to our neighbors that I can smell their laundry soap and dryer sheets.

I have to make myself go and do some things even if it makes me sick. If I don't do anything I feel depressed and it just eats at you and you end up getting worse. That's what happened to me when I didn't even go to the grocery store.

God has helped me through all of this. I'm a Catholic. I had lost my faith when my mother died back in 1981. But after I got sick I needed something to see me through and I went back to my religion. I pray to the Lord every day, all day long sometimes, to help me get through when I'm having a bad day. I used to go to Mass, but now it seems like there's more people going and I can't go. I've been going in the evenings but even then I get sick. I've been standing by the back door, and some of the ushers will keep the door open for me. The smell of perfume is still horrendous and I come out of there tasting it and with my body reeking of it. It attaches itself to me. I pray the whole time I'm in there to finish the Mass, but sometimes I come out of there ready to just scream and yell. I can't, because my daughter and my boyfriend would feel bad. They worry about me. So I go to my room to do my crying.

Some mornings I wake up crying. My family thinks it's because of them and they don't want to do anything to make me sick. They don't understand it's just the way my body reacts. I don't always even know what I'm reacting to. Sometimes I have a good week and I feel better, and then it all blows up in my face. I feel worse during the winter months. I don't know why. I try to put on a happy face all the time, but there are times when I wish I could just curl up and die. When you're feeling that bad everything looks negative.

Prayer helps me a lot. And I tell myself I'm just feeling bad and it will go away. I take a lot of vitamins, especially vitamin C. I give myself injections every three days, and once a month I get an IV. My former employer pays for all my medications and treatments. I don't know what I'll do if she ever stops.

I'm looking forward to making a pilgrimage to Chimayo this week. It's a pilgrimage people make for Easter every year. They walk to Chimayo from all over New Mexico and even farther. From Santa Fe it's an eight-hour walk. I did it once from here, but this year I'm not strong enough, so I'll start at the halfway point. People are very protective of me and don't want me to do it by myself. But I like to walk by myself so I can focus on my prayers. It's a long walk but very beautiful and cleansing.

Roy Bolbery
Santa Fe, New Mexico

A native of England, Roy Bolbery, forty-two when interviewed, was ill throughout his childhood in London. At age six he had a severe adverse reaction to penicillin. His sleep frequently was interrupted by night terrors. And during the day he would suddenly feel ill for no apparent reason. The outcome of many medical tests was a diagnosis of mild epilepsy. His sister died in childhood of leukemia. His father suffered with tuberculosis.

Born with a passion for automobiles and racing, Roy left school at age fifteen to study auto mechanics and engineering in a college program sponsored by the English government. He passed the program with flying colors and, still a teenager, went to work full-time as a certified automotive mechanic. Periods of illness with no apparent explanation continued to plague him in his work. He learned to accept this as a regular way of life. Beginning at the age of nineteen he was operating his own successful automotive repair business. Then a more glamorous opportunity came his way, and he went with a friend to work for Lotus, entertaining press, race car drivers and celebrities at European Grand Prix races. When the Grand Prix came to America, it was the golden opportunity Roy had been waiting for. At the conclusion of the racing season he stayed in the U.S., obtained a green card and went to work in a Beverly Hills sports car repair facility to work on Jaguars and Rolls-Royces. In 1980 he opened a specialty repair shop with two friends in Santa Fe, specializing in work on exotic cars. Eventually he and his partners parted company and Roy continued working on his own.

The event that changed his life and health occurred in March 1989, when he was painting shelves to move into a building he had just purchased as a workshop and live-in studio. The incident disabled him for several years.

Roy's creativity has enabled him to go back to work in the automotive industry in a way that won't further jeopardize his health. A warm and open individual, Roy addresses in this narrative the isolation he experiences and the difficulty of trying to create new relationships as a person with MCS.

My plan was to open a showroom for specialty cars, and I wanted this facility to look elegant. So, I painted some shelving with a special product which turned out to be deadly. Some friends had offered me the use of their industrial paint booth, with air filters and exhaust fans to suck out the fumes. Not wanting to inconvenience them, I declined the offer. I believed that I would be fine wearing a respirator and using an extractor fan in my old shop. I bought the paint and set to it, painting the shelves without a second thought. It was a big project that took me two days, on and off, to finish. By the time I finished I knew that something wasn't right. I felt extremely ill.

I went home and went to bed. After a short while I knew I had to see a doctor. It was all I could do to drag myself to my car and drive. I went to the hospital emergency room with the can of paint and explained what was happening to me. They pulled blood and made a vague attempt to call Poison Control in Albuquerque, but nobody had any information about the chemicals in the paint. Then they sent me home and told me to drink a lot of water. I went home expecting that I would start to feel better, but I didn't. My condition went downhill. My regular doctor didn't have any answers either, and so began the long battle.

Now, ten years later, I know that what was wrong with me was MCS. I've probably had chemical sensitivities all my life. I do know this exposure in 1989 put me on my deathbed. But back then hardly anyone spoke of MCS.

The financial commitment I'd just made to pur-

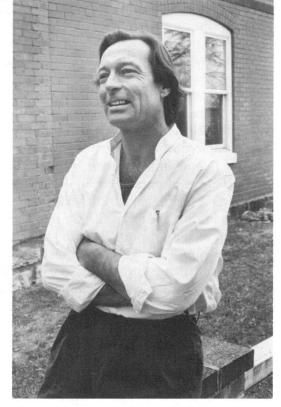

chase a building obviously compounded my stress. But in the beginning, not knowing what I was faced with, I assumed my condition would improve soon, and I could make the payments on the property. My credit was excellent, and I used credit cards to pay for medical bills and living expenses. I kept thinking surely by next week I'm going to feel better and I can get back to work and work my way out of this financial mess. But that day didn't come for years. I quickly ran up thirty thousand dollars in debt, and had to sell the building and close the business.

For a full year I was extremely ill, unable to function and, for the most part, alone. I think some of my closest friends didn't know what to do and they withdrew. My mother and her husband suggested I close my business and come to England. They promised they would help to get me back to Santa Fe when I was ready. I appreciated their offer of support, but I couldn't just let go of everything that for ten years I had worked so hard for. That was everything I had. Everything I knew. My survival. So I procrastinated on taking them up on their offer.

In a state of desperation, I went to see all kinds of different doctors, healers and alternative practitioners. Based on the symptoms I reported, one doctor told me I must have intestinal parasites. I was willing to go along with any glimmer of hope. I thought: If I have parasites, that can be treated, then my symptoms will go away—fantastic! However, I wanted a second opinion. I went to a doctor in Albuquerque who took urine, stool and saliva samples and sent them to a doctor in New York. The lab report said there were eggs from two kinds of parasites found, hookworm and whipworm. The doctor gave me herbal potions made from God-knows-what he had gathered in the rain forest. These remedies made me worse, so I decided to go to the Tropical Disease Hospital in London. It wasn't easy.

Going through the national health care program because I'm still a British subject entitled to benefits, I had to first see a family practitioner. I went to see my mother's doctor, about a hundred miles north of London. After I saw the doctor he wrote a letter to the hospital and was waiting to hear back by letter. It seemed ridiculous for me to sit around feeling like absolute hell, waiting for a letter. I felt like I was in a Third World country! I phoned the GP to tell him I was afraid for my life, and we needed to get the process expedited. I said, "Can't you fax the information and get this show on the road?" With that he contacted the hospital. When I finally went to my appointment they weren't interested in anything I said or any of the medical information I'd brought with me from America. And they found nothing, after testing me thoroughly. By then I didn't know if I had some parasite they didn't look for or if I'd been brainwashed in America.

In England the culture is quite different. You don't question a doctor's orders, and the doctor might not even tell you what your diagnosis is. Well, I was questioning everything because I was sick and no one could give me any explanation. I was angry with the doctors and anyone who told me to just go along with them. The GP had told the doctor in London I needed to see a psychiatrist. When my parents got word of that they didn't want to hear anything else. I said, "Look, it's not in my mind. This started when I got poisoned from the paint I was using. Something happened to me that day and I need to find out what it is. I'm losing my mind because no one has an explanation!"

By taking the whole situation into my own hands I was able to control my anger at the time. I came back to Santa Fe where access to the medical system and community was much easier than in England.

At one point I was referred to a doctor in Malibu, California, who wanted to see me three times a week because, according to him, I had fragmented and ulcerated gangrene around a part of my brain and was in the primary stages of developing a brain tumor. That news was devastating. He took several thousand dollars from me for the several visits I had with him and told me that I was being kept alive by angels. I quit going to him and had an MRI just to be on the safe side. And guess what—no brain tumor.

Another time a friend insisted I go to an appointment she'd made for me to see some kind of healer. Not knowing what I was getting into, I went and told the woman what had happened to me. What she told me was the most absurd thing I'd ever heard in my life. She said, "It's obvious that what has happened to you is that your exposure to the poison paint triggered memories of your most recent life when you were poisoned by mustard gas in World War I in the trenches of France."

Do I think a person like her, who can come up with such a far-fetched diagnosis of a situation, is arrogant and dangerous? Absolutely. A lot of people who are sick with MCS have been misled by charlatans. Therefore, the illness itself has been minimized and discounted.

Regardless of what anyone believes, I was exposed to toxic fumes from a paint gun in my hand and all of a sudden my life changed. It had to do with being poisoned by that product's poly-isocyonates.

I took information, piece by piece, and put together what has worked for me—lots of different techniques and approaches to healing and to life itself. I followed that path and got myself back to a place where I could function again. It wasn't until I started to improve, four years ago, that I became aware of my reactions when exposed to certain fumes—paints, aftershave, perfumes and other chemicals. Prior to that, I was so damned sick I didn't know chemical exposures were affecting me on such a major level.

What has helped me more than anything else is minimizing my exposure to chemicals in food, air and water. I've started eating organic foods and replaced all of my personal care and cleaning products with less-toxic, unscented products.

Friends who see me now often comment on how well I look. They've told me I used to look deathly ill. Every time they see me they ask me how I'm doing, because they realize how sick I've been and that I still don't always feel good. They understand that I can't be around people wearing fragrances, and that I can't go out just anywhere, and that when we do go out together I might have to move or leave suddenly. Whatever I have to do to protect myself is fine with them.

Three years ago I finally went back to work. I may be the only person with MCS on the planet who would go back to working in the automotive industry, but I do it in a manner that works fairly well for me. I've found nontoxic alternatives to the solvents and other chemicals I used to use, even for cleaning parts. I've put a radiant heat system in the ceiling so that I can have fresh air moving through the shop in the dead of winter and still be warm. Before I bring a car into my environment for work I always steam clean it. Any residual oil or gasoline on the engine is cleaned out, so I keep the fumes in my environment to a minimum. When draining oil I wear surgical gloves and coveralls and stay upwind of the fumes. Either I leave the shop until the oil has finished draining, or I wear a respirator. I also wear a respirator when I dispose of the old oil, fill the car with fresh oil, and seal it back up. I seem to be more affected by petroleum-based products, especially used engine oil, than by most other substances. Once in a while there is an unavoidable exposure that can knock me out for a couple of days if I'm not careful. I react in the same way to perfumes, which, interestingly, are petroleum-based.

My situation is less than ideal, but this is how I make my living. It isn't necessarily what I'm going to carry on doing. I have some other ideas that I may pursue.

Meanwhile, I've set up my shop so that I can control my air quality. I live next to the shop in an MCS-friendly motor home that I refurbished with safe materials. When I don't feel well I can go and rest. I'd be much better off if I didn't have to try to live a normal life, but I choose to do so. If I had the financial resources I would develop a commune for people with this condition. I'd love to know if such a place already exists, or if other people are thinking about this. That's the type of situation I hope to find in the future.

Because my work is not ideal for someone in my predicament, a certain part of me lives in fear of becoming unable to function again. I try to protect my health at all costs. My fear is that I couldn't survive.

Last winter I had a severe reaction to some waste oil. When I went to see my doctor he said I had pneumonia. When antibiotics had no effect I felt helpless. The doctor tested me again and said I had mono, which is caused by Epstein-Barr virus. This past winter I went to England for a visit, came back and went down with pneumonia again. Commercial air travel is a challenge for me because of poor air quality and unavoidable exposures to fragrances.

Another fear is that I won't ever find another life partner, which is something that I really want. I don't live what one would consider a normal life. It isn't normal. It isn't easy—far from it. With the exception of developing a relationship with a woman who has MCS, my options really are limited. I spend a lot of time alone, and that isn't what I want to do.

Trying to have a social life is terribly difficult because of my problem with fragrances. People who don't have the problem seem to have trouble grasping it. I've been involved in a couple of relationships since I've been sick. They didn't work out, at least partly because I'm not the easiest person to be with now because of my condition. That has been difficult for me. One of the things that has helped me to cope with the loss of relationships is a men's support group I participated in. That is something I never imagined I would try.

The fact of the matter is, I'm the one with the problem and I'm not going to change the world. I have to do whatever I can to improve my own environment, stay in it as much as I can, and protect myself when I leave my bubble. That's the best anyone can do. If I don't do that, I'm going to suffer.

A doctor in Dallas who has been treating me for the past year believes MCS may be a brain injury from chemicals, and put me on the drug Neurontin. Neurontin is an amino acid and was first used in the treatment of epilepsy—the diagnosis given to me as a child—so now I've come full circle. The Neurontin helped me a lot in the beginning, but then I had to increase the dose significantly to get the same effect. The drug is outrageously expensive. I am sponsored by a drug company, otherwise the cost would be prohibitive.

Ultimately, I see myself working with animals or helping people—maybe people with MCS in particular. I am considering applying to medical school in Cambridge, England, to study neurology.

On behalf of an MCS task force, I testified before the legislature here in Santa Fe and helped to raise funds for an MCS awareness program. It is imperative to educate the public about this condition. Helping to make that happen feeds me on an emotional and spiritual level.

If nothing else, this illness has enabled me to really get to know myself and has taken me down pathways I may never have found otherwise.

Jennifer
Santa Fe, New Mexico

Jennifer, twenty-seven when we spoke, is one of many chemically sensitive people who have moved to Santa Fe in desperation. Before she made the move she was so reactive to everything in her indoor environment that for four years in Colorado she lived outside as much as she possibly could without freezing. A native of Minnesota, she was a freshman at Colorado College when she became disabled at age nineteen. Instead of living the life she had dreamed of as an independent college coed, she has been an invalid throughout most of her twenties. The hardest part of coping with her illness has been missing out on all the "normal" activities of this stage of life.

Jennifer has a long history of allergies, injuries and physical problems that all seem to overlap, and a family history of environmental illness. Her grandmother had a lot of allergies and her mother is sensitive to perfume and cigarette smoke. Her brother became sensitive to chemicals while working in a lab with toxic waste, and now is extremely "allergic" to perfume. As a child Jennifer often had allergy "shiners" under her eyes, although no one realized that that was what they were at the time. When her tonsils were removed her reactions to anesthetics and medications kept her hospitalized for two weeks. In the sixth grade she developed problems with her connective tissue and digestive system. She lost twenty pounds, gave up gymnastics and used crutches for a year, then went back to sports.

In high school she developed an eating disorder and pushed her body to its limits in long-distance running, skiing, tennis, cycling and other sports. She also led wilderness backpacking and canoe trips.

In college she was training hard every day, eating poorly and sacrificing sleep to study and party. Her body finally gave out. A groin injury crippled her completely. After surgery it wouldn't heal and she was confined to a bed for three years. Since then her health has been further compromised by a series of events. At one point she developed a staph infection when her appendix was removed. The infection didn't show up until two years later when her navel began to ooze after a massage. Seven years later, it still oozes. She is now treating it with homeopathy because surgery is considered too risky for her.

Quite by accident Jennifer discovered that her tendon and connective tissue problems and chronic fatigue were exasperated by molds and chemical exposures. Her understanding is that her various health problems are related to but not completely caused by MCS. One doctor's theory is that her MCS and connective tissue problems may be caused by a metabolic dysfunction. Another doctor, after looking at her extensive medical history, told her she will never find an answer. Jennifer summarizes her ten years of medical tests and examinations by saying that her body doesn't absorb nutrients and her immune system has collapsed.

Jennifer requested that her last name not be published in order to protect her privacy.

My first year of college was the best year of my life, until I became so crippled I couldn't even walk. I had a lot of jobs and led a lot of wilderness trips to the Boundary Waters in Minnesota. Actually, I was hyperactive, which can be a symptom of allergies.

All my jobs were very physical, and I had a series of injuries that year. I had surgery for a groin injury, and it wouldn't heal. I went to numerous doctors and pain clinics, and finally went to Mayo Clinic for a month, where they put me on muscle relaxers, pain killers, steroids and twelve Advil a day. None of that made much of a difference, and probably set me up for my environmental illness. I was in such severe pain that I couldn't sit or walk. We had no idea what was wrong.

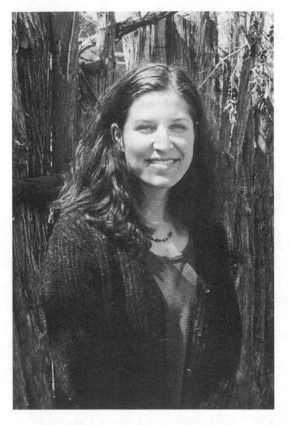

I was so sick of going to doctors that I didn't want to go to another one, but my mom took me to an osteopath who discovered my hips were severely out of place. He moved them back into place and my health began to improve. But by that time my system was so depleted, I was still confined to my bed or wheelchair and didn't get any exercise.

That winter the whole inside of my parents' house was painted with an oil-based paint. After that my tendons swelled, I had to wear a neck brace and I couldn't even feed myself, but we didn't realize there was a connection between the chemical exposure and my health. The tendons in my eyes were so swollen I could hardly see. It was terrifying and traumatic for me. For three years I was in bed, couldn't see anybody or do anything. It was all I could do to try to sit for a few minutes at a time. I missed my friends from college, missed school and missed my active life. I wasn't in touch with my feelings at the time. I had to stay above them or I never would have survived.

The only kind of therapy I could do was in a heated pool. They would put me in the water right in my wheelchair, and a therapist would help me to move a little bit. I did that three times a week, until we realized that I was chemically sensitive. Then I discontinued the water therapy to minimize my chemical exposures. Prior to that, I also started seeing alternative doctors who found I was depleted in all kinds of nutrients. They put me on amino acids and gave me IV vitamins but still hadn't made the environmental connection.

To give my mother a break from caretaking me twenty-four hours a day, I went to stay with a friend of the family whose husband was away. This woman used all fragrance-free and nontoxic products because she was slightly sensitive to chemicals. A couple days after I moved into her house I could walk a little, and in a few weeks I was much better. That's how I finally realized that chemical exposures were affecting my health. At first I was excited because I thought that I would completely recover by changing my diet and lifestyle. I read a lot about MCS and environmental illness, and my doctor started helping me to detoxify my body. I ended up living with our friend for nine months and improved a lot. But I've also learned that doctors have never seen some of my symptoms in others with environmental illness, so part of my problems seem to be something separate, and I continue to see other specialists.

I've been told that my environmental illness and connective tissue problems may be partly caused by a metabolic problem. I'm not getting nutrients to where I need them in my body. This year it's starting to affect the collagen of my skin.

One metabolic specialist I saw looked at my medical records and said, "You're not going to find answers." We'd spent thousands of dollars and I was still sick. She asked me what I'd done that had helped, and I told her I ate organic foods and avoided chemical exposures. She told me to keep doing that, which was amazing to me. I don't usually mention my chemical sensitivities to mainstream doctors.

That spring I took a turn for the worse because I was reacting to molds and pesticides. On top of that, our friend's husband, who doesn't believe in environmental illness, came home, and he wore a heavy scent. My body just collapsed again with chronic fatigue. That time I was in bed again four months, unable to do anything.

When my doctor realized that I was extremely sensitive to mold he told me to go back to Colorado where it was drier. As soon as I was strong enough to sit, I got on a plane and went to Colorado, rented a room in the house owned by a wonderful woman named Ruth who led an MCS support group. She said she's never seen anyone as sick as I was, and she helped me a lot. But her house was so moldy that I got even worse and had to sleep outside. That was the start of living outside on and off for four years because I never could find housing that didn't make me worse. I had such a hard time in Colorado that I don't care if I ever go back to that state again.

My mom brought out all my things and wound up staying for four months trying to find housing for me. Part of the time she stayed in cabins and part of the time she camped with me, even though she hates to camp. I had to use a blue plastic tarp to make an A-frame for myself, because even tents were making me sick. Out of desperation we looked for a house to buy, even though we couldn't afford it. We looked way up in the mountains and all over Colorado, but nothing worked for me.

One October was so cold I needed to be inside, so we took a cabin knowing it was not a good place for me. We tried to make it safer by covering the whole thing in foil. My mom and I foiled all the floors, the walls and even the furniture. But I was still reacting. A friend of mine with MCS came to try to help me figure out what was causing the problem. It was a mystery. The X factor. Then I realized I was reacting to the foil! I was also reacting to the electromagnetic fields. So we covered all the foil with tapestries. We called it the "hippie" house. I got really sick in there but I had to stay for the winter. There was nothing else.

That spring I was coming to Santa Fe for medical treatments. I used hand controls to drive my car without using my legs and feet all the time. That gave me more freedom, but sometimes I was so sick that Ruth or another friend had to drive me, or my mom would have to come from Minnesota to go with me. I gave the treatments a good shot, but they only made me worse and I gave that up after a year and a half.

The summer after I stayed in that cabin was my "summer from hell." I was twenty-two. All my life I'd felt invincible, and now I couldn't even fully take care of myself, though I desperately wanted to. I tried to stay at Ruth's house again and got so sick from the mold that I couldn't move. My mother had to fly out, with hardly any notice, to get me out of the house. She wound up camping with me in national parks most of that summer. I couldn't have done it without her.

My mother has gone through hell with this. She and my father have spent their retirement funds on my health care. I don't know what they'll do when they retire. This has been so difficult for my mother, she's gone through some counseling just to help her cope. She deserves so much credit. She has scrubbed walls, cleaned carpets and foiled condos or cabins, trying to make them safe for me, only to find out it wouldn't work, and start all over again in another place. She really got worried when my brother developed chemical sensitivities when he was working as a chemist in a toxic lab. He looked horrid, and my mother was so worried. She said, "We can't afford another one!" He left that job and now works outside as a hydro-geologist, and he looks great. But he's still very sensitive to fragrances.

A boyfriend from college also supported me through those years in Colorado, especially one winter when I was living in an isolated cabin. He brought me things I needed and kept me company on the weekends. We spent a lot of time talking. He hiked while I rested. He did things for me that I couldn't do myself, like vacuum the floors and take out the trash. Those are the kinds of things I still can't do, so I have arranged for my roommates to take care of those things.

I experienced a lot of fiascoes while I was living outside. One time a bear came into my campsite because my cooler was sitting on the ground. I knew from my wilderness experience that it wasn't safe to leave food or coolers on the ground, but I didn't have a choice. I was physically unable to stash my cooler in a tree. The bear threw the cooler around and pawed through the food, then came and sniffed all over me while I lay still in my sleeping bag. I couldn't move. There was nothing I could do but lay quietly and pray. The bear finally left about an hour later. My food was strewn all over the ground and there was nothing I could do about it. My mother wasn't coming back until the next afternoon. By noon the next day I was so hungry that I stuck my hand into a jar that was dripping with bear saliva and ate some of the spoiled food. The cooler survived—which I always thought would have made a good Coleman commercial!

That was when there were only about nine foods I could eat, mostly plain meat and vegetables. I'd go to a friend's house or my mom's cabin to steam enough vegetables to eat for four days.

Another close call was when I was camping alone, way out in a deserted campground and a creepy guy came along. I was never so scared in my life. My mother was gone with the car and not coming back until the next day. There was no place to hide and no way to get away. I just kept saying, "My mother will be here soon." I lucked out and he left me alone.

I didn't tell my mother about the incident right away because I didn't want her to worry. But I decided that from then on I would camp in more populated areas. The problem with that, though, was that I had to move several times a day and several times a night because I'd get wind from a camp fire or somebody using bug spray.

When my mother was sick of camping out she would stay in

a cabin or condo. There were times when she had to drive out and try to find me in the dark when it was storming, because she knew the wind and rain would blow my tarp away, and that I was too weak to recover it myself. She'd find me, find my tarp and stake it down again.

Trying to find a place to shower was another challenge when I was homeless. Sometimes I found showers in office buildings. Quite often I showered in a building where I went for body work. Or I would go to a friend's, or to the cabin or condo where my mother was staying, just long enough to take a quick shower.

One time my mother was staying in a cabin at a campground, and the maintenance crew had just cleaned out the water pipes with chlorine. I didn't know it, but all the other campers were complaining because they'd used too much chlorine and it had caused a toxic hazard. I went in and took a shower, thinking the chlorine smelled strong to me because I was so sensitive. My mother walked in and screamed, "Get out of the shower! That's pure chlorine they're dumping on you!" By then my skin and hair were saturated with chlorine, and I had to get it out. I remembered a massage therapist who had said I could come to her place if I ever needed a shower or bath. So, at ten o'clock at night my mother and I arrived at her door, freezing cold, and this sweet woman took us in. It was a most magical night I will always remember because it had been so long since I'd had a hot bath, and my mom got to sit with the family enjoying hot tea and cookies and watching a movie.

Another memorable shower incident happened when I went to get a haircut. Before I could stop the woman she sprayed some detangler or something on my hair. I was extraordinarily sensitive to everything at the time and it made me horribly sick. I had to get it out. So, my mother and I went to my friend's house but she couldn't let us in because the smell of the hair product made her sick, too. So my mother tried to wash my hair with vinegar and baking soda outside with the garden hose. Then we started driving back to my campground, an hour away. We were both tired and ornery and wanted to sleep. But the smell was still on my hair and making me sick. I tried to cover it up with a cap, and that didn't work either. As much as I hated to I said, "Mom, we've got to go back to Lisa's to get out this smell." We drove back, I took off my clothes, covered my body with plastic garbage bags and drenched my hair outside with tomato juice. We knew that tomato juice takes away the skunk smell from dogs that have been sprayed. We figured that if it worked for that it would work on this hair product. All the neighbors must have wondered what in the world I was doing outside in the freezing snow with plastic bags on me! It did work, but I remember freezing the rest of that night.

When I was so exhausted from living outside I tried to live in Estes Park, where I'd be close to my doctor appointments. I relied on body work—and still do—to keep my body functioning. But the place I moved to didn't work at all. That's when I called an environmentally ill woman I'd heard about in Santa Fe and asked her if I could rent a room in her house. It was a stab in the dark. I couldn't believe it when she said yes. I lived like a recluse in that house on a lake twenty minutes out of town. Came into town for doctor appointments several times a week. That's when I really started to get well. I think it helped me enormously to have a stable, safe place to live for the first time in years. I also started a new treatment program, doing a lot of energy work.

Within four months I could tolerate almost anything. I felt so good that I was going out to bars and movies. I quit eating organic foods and got really hyper again. I even interviewed for a secretarial job, thinking I could work at least part-time. I separated from my boyfriend because I realized I needed to date other people because I had missed out on so much. I rented an apartment closer to town to make it easier to meet with friends, and my mother moved all my belongings. After a year of dating and not taking good care of myself, my body crashed again. All my old symptoms came back and now I can't go near a store without feeling sick from the smells—which I couldn't even smell when I was feeling well.

I've had to learn to mask my symptoms to a point so that I can even function in the world. There is such a fine line between masking a little bit so it doesn't hurt your health, and masking so much that it does hurt your health. When I was going to bars, I masked way too much and it really hurt me.

This past year I developed a whole series of infections and wasn't functioning at all. I never told my folks, but the doctors were quite seriously worried about my condition. They put me on a lot of antifungal, antiviral and antibacterial drugs, which weren't really good for me but they didn't have a choice. I was wasting away. My spine was affected, I got a slipped disk, and had to wear a neck brace and stay in bed for months.

Fortunately, my MCS doesn't cause me to feel depressed like it does a lot of people. I'll get depressed if I think about my situation too much, but anyone with any illness is going to feel worse if they think about the illness twenty-four hours a day. I try not to focus on it too much, and I only talk about it with a few close friends. The only people I associate with are people with positive attitudes. Even when I'm with friends who have MCS, we don't talk much about our illness. We talk about life. I love books, so I talk about books. I rent a lot of movies, so I talk about those. I'm interested in spiritual issues, and I tend to pick friends who are spiritual too, so we talk about that. I like taking a class because that gives me something interesting to do and to talk about, too. We share information about things that have worked for us, and we laugh together.

A part of me lives in a chronic state of fear, though. When my back went out I was afraid of what it might mean. Would I be in bed for two months or two days? Some of my other fears are financial. Will I lose my disability? Will I have to move back to my parents' house? Another fear I have is that my neighbor will use pesticides. I will have to leave my house if she does.

I've had to learn to manage my fears about going to places where I've gotten sick from chemical exposures before. Toxins do make you sick, so you learn to be afraid of them, especially when your illness is really severe. When I think about how ill I've been or how close I've come to passing out in a place before, I'm sure to feel sick when I go in again. But if I don't think about it and just go in to do what I need to do, I might be okay or I might have to leave, depending on the environment and my tolerance that day. My friends do the same thing to survive.

You have to monitor the fear or you sacrifice your quality of life. A lot of people wouldn't want me to say that, because people who don't have MCS might think that means the illness is just something caused by the fear. But that isn't true. What I mean is that fear can reduce what quality of life we do have. You have to find out what you *can* do. You have to live. You have to do things or you're going to wither away inside, and that's not going to help your health.

Acceptance is something else that I'm working on. My spiritual director has suggested that I hang around positive people who have disabilities, to help me learn to accept mine. A person who is quadriplegic or paralyzed knows their limitations right off. They spend the first year or two accepting their limitations and then they move on. I've never been able to accept or move on because I don't know what my limitations are going to be in the future. I may be this way the rest of my life. I hate to even think that, because there are so many things I want to do that require more strength than I have now. I've accepted that I'm not ever going to climb Mt. Everest; I'm not ever going to be that physical. All I really want to do is to be able to hike again. I've given up on backpacking. Just going for a walk would be nice.

When you've had a chronic illness for years, like I have, it becomes a way of life and you can get stuck in that pattern. I'm working on that now. I use various alternative therapies to move those patterns out of my memory and body. Rubenfeld is my favorite. It gets you grounded in your body. Emotionally I've left my body because it's in so much pain that I don't want to be in it.

My physical problems also are worsened because I don't feel my emotions very well, so I'm working hard on that level too. I believe that any illness has an emotional component. The illness can either start at the emotional level and cause physical problems, or start at the physical level and cause emotional distress. I don't think it really matters where it started, in order to heal you have to work on every level. I'm so cut off from my emotions because that's what I've had to do to survive what I've gone through. Now I'm learning to allow myself to feel my feelings even when they're painful.

I'm extremely sensitive to stress and other people's emotional energy. It's like I have radar. I think that's part of my problem. I was always sensitive as a child, but I didn't realize how sensitive. Right now it's a detriment because I turn it inward and can't turn it off. But it's a gift that I'm trying to develop in a positive direction.

I have to have roommates who are low-keyed, and who are willing to accommodate me. I've learned to screen them pretty well. Males are easier to live with than females, for me, because guys don't seem to care what kind of soap or shampoo they use. I just hand it to them and they think, "This is great, it's free!"

I don't want to act neurotic about my illness or scare potential roommates off, so I just tell them I'm somewhat sensitive to chemicals and fragrances, and they will have to use natural products. A lot of roommates have ended up smoking, so I have to be careful to screen for that now. And this year I've developed more spine problems, so I need more help around the apartment. I offer to take twenty bucks a month off the rent if they will do the things that I can't do, like vacuum and mop the floors, lift the plants and take out the trash. I clean the kitchen, dust and do whatever I can.

Sometimes I feel embarrassed about how much time I spend in bed or watching TV. I used to hate TV, but now I watch it when I'm too tired to read and my brain just doesn't work. It's also difficult when people ask me what I do. People who aren't sick don't realize I have to do things to take care of my health all day.

I can't give up. I'm only twenty-seven and I have a whole life ahead of me. Giving up has never been an option.

I'm dreaming of getting a master's degree in counseling. Lately I've been wondering if I'll ever be able to work on a degree that intensely, but that's what I really want to do. I've had so many kinds of treatment that I know the difference between a good practitioner and a bad one, a great one from a good one. Right now I'm taking one class at a time.

The most important lesson I've learned is to really feel and experience my emotions. That's what brings happiness and joy. And when it feels like there is no joy, I know that feeling will pass. My friends say I'm going to be a very happy, well-adjusted adult, despite the fact that I've missed out on my twenties.

Susan Molloy
Snowflake, Arizona

Duality is part of life with MCS. This phenomenon is particularly striking in the life of Susan Molloy, a petite woman with a larger-than-life personality, known across the country for her MCS advocacy. Due to the severity of her reactions to chemicals and electromagnetic fields (EMFs), first impressions of Susan vary dramatically, depending on where you meet her.

Those who encounter her in EMF- and chemically-polluted environments see a woman strapped to a wheelchair, unable to articulate clearly, sometimes breathing from an oxygen tank, and wearing an old army helmet to protect herself. Strangers often assume she is severely developmentally impaired with cerebral palsy, and wouldn't dream she is a competent martial artist.

In a safe environment her presence is radiating. She can walk, run and talk a blue streak. At her home in a remote location near Snowflake, Arizona, I experienced her as articulate, intelligent, feisty, playful and warm.

Susan's is one of nine households of chemically sensitive people who have clustered in the desert near Snowflake, seeking respite from the pollutants of more populated areas and creating their own safe community. One family, their health greatly improved, recently moved on to Montana to resume a more mainstream lifestyle. Susan and one other EI neighbor woman are members of the Unitarian-Universalist Church, despite the fact they cannot attend traditional services. The two women meet in Susan's home or talk on the phone.

Living on less than five hundred dollars a month from Social Security income, Susan recently became the owner of a small home built to meet her environmental needs. The kitchen, living and work areas are all part of one open room. Electrical equipment is limited to a computer and television, both carefully sealed and shielded to minimize EMF exposures.

It didn't occur to me until after I'd left that I had been oblivious to EMF issues. Arriving with a tape recorder operating on electricity showed my lack of awareness, as did my confusion when Susan inspected my equipment before allowing me to use an outlet. The purpose of her inspection eluded me until I'd heard her story, driven away and allowed the reality to sink in. Then I felt like a blundering idiot. Now that my consciousness is raised regarding EMF sensitivity, I will always be prepared to operate my recorder on batteries when appropriate. The upshot is that, for the first time in twenty years of recording interviews, my equipment malfunctioned and much of the interview had not recorded. Was this a coincidence, or did the recorder fail due to an upset of some delicate electromagnetic balance? We'll never know. I chalked it up to bizarre coincidence and recaptured the interview by telephone. Oddly enough, even the tapes from the telephone conversations produced unusual sounds.

Born and raised in Oregon and on the north coast of California, Susan and her family moved often due to her father's work in the lumber industry, overseeing the development of the first particleboard plants in the U.S. During summers as a child she worked in fields, picking—and eating—fruits and vegetables freshly sprayed with pesticides. Although she experienced abnormal reactions at the time, she never connected those with toxic contamination.

As a student at San Francisco State University, Susan was a political activist during the Vietnam era. While on hiatus from school she traveled extensively in Southeast Asia, Europe and Central America. During that time she received numerous inoculations and used DEET-containing insect repellents daily on her body, hair and clothing. Now she wonders if that relates to the onset of her severe chemical reactions approximately one year after she returned to the U.S. in the early '80s.

Susan completed her undergraduate work at the University of California at Berkeley, followed by training and work as a paralegal. Later, in spite of serious chemical and electromagnetic field barriers, she earned a master's degree in disability policy. A divorce was one of the challenges she faced during that chapter of her life.

Susan's name now is synonymous with MCS accommodations in California and beyond. She was instrumental in the development of an environmentally-friendly wing in the Marin County hospital; the development of an experimental, eleven-unit apartment house funded by the government for people with MCS, also in Marin County; and a designated fragrance-free area in a Unitarian Church in San Francisco.

As a founder of the National Coalition for the Chemically Injured, much of her current work is at the national level.

This disease hurts in the oddest ways. Whether you lose a lot all at once—your job, your house and your family—or over a period of time, like flesh being picked from your bones by a cruel slow bird, you feel a certain amount of envy or jealousy toward people who still have all the toys, still have all the flesh on their bones. I sometimes feel jealous of my own colleagues, or people on a similar path, who can afford medical care or who easily obtain safe housing and things like that. However, every time I'm stricken hard with jealousy or envy, I've been privileged to be shown the situation up close, and that dispels the feelings, because nothing is as simple as it first appears. Someone who has access to medical treatments that I can't afford might be made worse. Or the person with the loyal, supportive spouse or partner may have other kinds of problems I don't have.

There is no real safety with this illness. There are no rules, no teacher, you don't know where the bottom is. My favorite coping strategy is studying karate and tae kwon do, where there are rules, there is safety, there is a teacher, and I can defend myself. There is physical pain, when I make an error, but it is without fear.

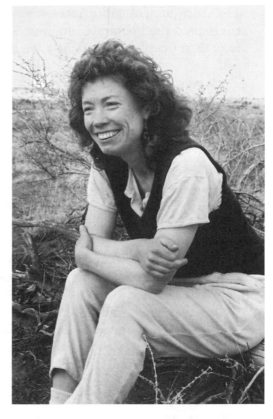

The part of me that feels most blessed is the part that's oblivious to interior decor and four-course dinners. I don't need to shop at Bloomingdale's or Nordstrom's. It's okay to live here in my bunker at plain little "Camp Snowflake." It's pretty enough, and I'm strong here so I can take care of myself and help people with their projects.

The first time an emergency room doc told me I was having an allergic reaction, in 1981, I didn't believe it. I didn't like people with allergies and I had the usual prejudices against people who were hypersensitive. It sounded very unlikely to me that those doctors were right. I didn't want to have allergies. But I was in a terrifying medical situation. My throat and palate and sinuses had swelled closed and I had hives all over my body. The hives became urticaria, which means fluids rapidly leak from the cells in your body into the wrong places, and you go into shock. I became swollen and unable to breathe within a few minutes, and I felt such panic. My life was saved repeatedly in emergency rooms, and the doctors kept saying I was having allergic reactions.

One of the things that frightened me the most about the reaction is how fast it comes on. Within minutes my lips can puff up and my eyes can swell shut. My face can look like a monster's. It's very frightening when you don't know what's going on. It frightened me, and it frightened cab drivers who took me to the hospitals and it frightened the hospitals' employees. Eventually I got bee sting kits to give to people, to keep me alive long enough so I could get to the ER.

I started keeping a notebook to try to figure out what was causing these reactions. It turned out to be various foods, cigarette smoke, cleansers, mold, vehicle exhaust, pesticides, cosmetics, soap, my clothes and electromagnetic fields.

I was experiencing panic and fear, which I feel was justified. I had to become someone who managed the behavior of other people, to some degree, to keep myself alive, a very uncomfortable position to be in. I found myself having to ask people to not smoke or not to use personal care products or cleaning products. That was mortifying. I didn't want to care what other people did. It is philosophically offensive to have to care about such trivia. I didn't know anyone else with this disease, so I didn't have a model on which to base the behavior I was having to exercise. On the other hand, the reactions were swift and violent and I didn't have much choice.

I could feel and sense input from all manner of environmental elements and food and so forth. At the time I had no context for what was happening, and felt quite mad. Some of what I considered madness at the time was actually my having been acutely perceptive and acutely accurate about what I felt and sensed. Those of us with chemical and electromagnetic field sensitivities have extra senses. I have no way to accurately describe these to people who have never experienced it. It is a true advantage in many respects, but it's weird being that odd person who can sense trouble—that the power lines are leaking or the gas line is leaking.

My friends realized I was in horrible trouble and, with the best of intentions I'm sure, they made a plan to have me committed to a mental health facility. One friend recognized that the exposures and food in hospital would mean my death, and told me about the planned "intervention" at the last second. He knew I was not in good shape and that I could not take care of myself, and I knew it, too. At least he recognized I didn't belong in a mental health facility, for which I am forever grateful. I guess there were arguments about letting me slip away, but no one is sorry now. I stayed with different sets of friends for a while and then with my parents in Northern California.

Thank God for my family. They really came through. They had

to change tremendously in order to keep me alive. We went through three winters without being able to use any heat, and they couldn't cook the foods they were used to. My mother collected rain and bottled it for me. And my dad got to be a really good emergency driver, a real ace. It took him sitting with me through a real bad ER visit after a pesticide exposure, when I nearly died, before he fully understood the severity of my condition. The doctors explained to him what was going on and how to take care of me.

Family dynamics can change radically when one member has a sickness and disability and needs a lot of care. It was difficult for all of us. My relationship with them had been one of rebellion and defiance, typical for a precocious teenager in the '60s and a 20-year-old in the '70s. I didn't want to share their house or their values, but there I was, completely dependent on them again, and they were pretty much stuck with me in this condition. There was nothing to do but submit to this "child" role. I didn't know if I'd get well or not, but I felt stronger after a couple of years, and that had to be good enough. I stayed with my parents for almost three years.

I went through real fits and starts adjusting to this disease. Any coping skills on which I had relied before were certainly not available after I became sick. I was unnerved by this illness and by looking peculiar to people. My credibility seemed altered as responses from other people were so different from what I had experienced previously. Any self-esteem I had was shot to heck. Even though under certain circumstances I'm vulnerable, I do not want to be a wimp. That's not who I am. Now I know a lot of women with MCS who have real integrity, real loyalty and real love for their families and people for whom they are responsible. They never wimped out— they held on until the last minute. They took it as long as they could.

In 1985, I finally took the county public health psychiatrist's recommendation to try Desipramine, an ostensibly "mild" tricyclic antidepressant. I took tiny dot doses, and for a month or so I felt encouraged except for intense muscle tension and clenching. The psychiatrist said it was not remotely possible that this response was related to the medication. I took a low dose for four more months before throwing them out. The side effects had escalated horribly, and become what I later learned are called tardive dyskinesia and tardive dystonia. Subsequently, chemical and electromagnetic field exposures, feeling compromised or ashamed, or stress can trigger uncontrollable movement, hyperactivity, rigid posture and then, frequently, paralysis.

My motor control is impaired and my speech is impaired when I am exposed to chemicals and EMFs. I experience contorted movement and my muscles contract. I look, move and talk like I have cerebral palsy. My speech is unintelligible to some people. At one point walking outside became so difficult that I couldn't get across a street or close to major power lines without falling down. I had to dodge underground power lines in San Francisco and the streets connected to BART [Bay Area Rapid Transit]. It was the most unlikely situation. At that point a person really wonders what in the world to do with one's body. I used a wheelchair for many years, so I could go out in spite of the electrical transformers and still manage. Now I sometimes wear a metal World War II army helmet for working on the computer, or walking or driving under power lines, or going into buildings with low ceilings and fluorescent lighting. The helmet has a high iron content, and it's protective against some magnetic fields. I manage without the helmet in a gymnasium or someplace with very high ceilings, because it isn't the fluorescent flicker that makes me sick, it's the magnetic field from the ballast.

When I first began to experience the reactions in 1981, I tried to protect myself by covering my hands and feet. I wore several layers of cotton socks and an old plastic bag over each foot, and then galoshes. I covered my hands with cotton gloves and then surgical gloves for doing chores or going to the market. It did enable me to get around for a few weeks, but the repercussion was that a fungus grew on my feet and hands. It infected the nail bed of all my nails for a couple of years. It was ugly and frightening and my nails looked like the talons of a bird, black and yellow and very thick and hooked over. They were so thick I couldn't cut them. I heard horror stories that the nails needed surgical removal, or my toes and fingers needed amputation. Curing that wretched, disgusting fungus on my hands and feet was accomplished by my mother and cost approximately three dollars. She used a large kettle, a gallon of rainwater, and a bark from the South American Pau d'Arco tree. The bark was suggested by a friend of hers who used it to prevent mold growth on plants. They put a generous handful of the bark into a kettle and cooked it hard for an hour. Then, with the syrupy liquid, we were able to cure the fungus in two weeks—which I found pretty impressive. The nails grew right out. All the new growth was pink. The cuticles were intact and my fingers worked again. The talons grew off and haven't been back since. That was about 1984.

Early on, I went to two meetings of a support group called the Environmental Illness Association in San Francisco. I was intrigued to meet other people who had health problems that were somewhat similar to mine. The strangeness of their symptoms was frightening, but their coping strategies were provocative. Hearing their stories and the accommodations they had accomplished meant an awful lot to me. Some of the people in the meeting were professional people with very normal jobs and lives. One who impressed me was a woman from Palo Alto, and another was a fellow who worked in the financial district in San Francisco. It was helpful to me to see that businessmen and dentists and people who wore pearls could get this disease—all sorts of people from every class. I remember the relief of realizing this disease wasn't something I'd brought on myself by traveling too much, or participating in demonstrations, or being the "wrong" person or doing the "wrong" things. Sometimes the thought still surfaces that somehow I got sick because I felt so much political anger and social sorrow after Reagan was elected and many social services programs were dismantled. It felt like being sick had something to do with poor morale and the desperate way I felt about the direction our country was going. I couldn't get out and protest anymore, I couldn't help refugees, I couldn't send money to people who needed it. I felt inadequate and inept. There was a lot of sadness, a lot of sorrow. It was absolutely astonishing to me to meet Republicans at the support group who had this disease. I could hardly believe it.

Very soon after going to that support group I knew I needed to work on a political direction. We had what seemed to me to be a disabling condition, and we were not being accommodated, with housing, for example. I didn't have the language, or the legal terminology, or the disability policy background at that point, but I knew that's what I had to work on. People with chemical sensitivities or chemical injury are held to an absolutely absurd standard in terms of having to prove the etiology of the disease. I wanted to put some time and energy into helping people with that part of our experience that requires political expression.

A few years into my recovery I moved back to Marin County and was married. I wanted to have kids and have a job. I was aiming for "normal." But I was unable to stay pregnant longer than a couple of weeks. At the San Francisco General Hospital fertility clinic I learned that I seemed to create an immune reaction that stopped pregnancy. Fortunately, I've been able to live with other people's kids and care for them. There are always people around who have more kids than patience, so I can borrow kids.

In Marin I ran into situations time and again when someone I knew couldn't enter the hospital because there was new carpet, or couldn't get a pap smear or a breast exam, or couldn't take kids to the ER or to a clinic because of chemical barriers. I began working with some of the disability activists in Marin County and San Francisco and tried to learn what the laws were. In 1985 I started a newsletter, called *The Reactor*, about civil rights and access rights for people with chemical and electric magnetic field sensitivities.

Eventually I needed to go back to college to reorganize my talents and skills so they would better suit my "new" body and my new perspective on what was needed. I applied to three grad schools, but after I visited the campuses I realized I couldn't survive going as far as Berkeley or San Jose. Being trapped in traffic jams for hours a day on an oxygen tank and not being able to walk was too frightening.

I was admitted to San Francisco State University, which was closer, to the Department of Public Administration. I was able to find a wonderful faculty advisor there who said, "I don't really understand what you're telling me about your access needs, but I intuit that you're right and I will help you." She stuck with me for five years until I graduated with a degree in disability policy. It was truly hard, and I'm not sure it was a good idea to have done it. The environmental exposures were devastating. It was brutal going in and out of buildings for those five years, and coping with the prejudices of the faculty and other students. I had to keep an A-average throughout the five years because my disability required so much accommodation from the school and other people in the classrooms that I had to prove myself time after time after time.

One of my professors—who turned out to be a true favorite— wouldn't call on me for the first several weeks of our seminar. I think he was put off by having someone spastic and or paralyzed in his graduate economics seminar. It was hard for him to come to grips with issues such as whether or not I was thinking inside that body. I was paralyzed and drooling and couldn't look him in the eye. I couldn't articulate ideas except at home, in writing, and his prejudice and my self-consciousness got in our way. I worked real hard in that class, and he wound up being a supportive friend. It required a lot of growth on both our parts—me to have enough guts to stay with that class even through his distaste and my fear, and not knowing how to care for myself properly.

The physical disability is tiring but manageable. I know how to get strapped into the wheelchair. I know where the curb cuts are and how to maneuver the chair. I can cope with the industrial respirator. If I have to wear my army helmet I can do that, too, although I hate to in public places because who wants to look like a geek? But sometimes that's what I have to do. I know how to use oxygen effectively.

What makes me upset is that I crumble emotionally, or I'll have a flare of temper that can be triggered by an exposure or by some particularly demanding event. Behavioral and emotional stability are sadly lacking at times, and that's what I miss the most.

In my house or in my own yard where I have safe air I can defend and care for myself and my household and act like an adult. When I'm out in public places I need a lot of assistance and I don't feel confident.

What enabled me to persevere in grad school? The only part of the answer of which I'm very sure is that I couldn't find anyone in a position of responsibility or authority to help us. It seemed that somebody better start organizing what strength we have to work on projects and get some successes, some respect. The lawmakers and people who run hospitals and schools and businesses don't have enough courage to take a risk and help us unless they see us being potentially successful.

It seemed important to learn the language of government, and to start to work on housing programs for us and enabling non-profit groups to get funding to work toward accessible clinics and things like that. I just couldn't find anybody else to do it. I don't want to wind up incapacitated in a conventional nursing home. That means somebody is going to have a lot of work to do to get housing and accessible medical care established for people with chemical sensitivities and related disabilities. We can do it—it's going to require ongoing efforts to somehow make an effective bridge between those of us with this disability and the policymakers. The political work needs to be done in the most desperate way.

Our advocacy to date has often resulted in research projects. We've gotten some acknowledgment by the Social Security and Veterans' Administrations and Housing and Urban Development, the

Department of Justice and some of the larger federal and state agencies, but, typically, in name only. We don't have enforceable policies yet to protect us. We don't have fallbacks of unions or pension funds. We don't have real protection. That's humbling and it makes me angry.

I live for those hours each week in my martial arts class when I get to break boards. It helps counter the way I feel the rest of the time. I carry so much pent up anger and pain from the hundreds of times that people have jeopardized my life and my safety by their behavior, and kicking is an outlet. Some people can find that outlet through prayer. For me, it takes prayer and breaking some boards— hours of forceful, physical exercise, when I'm not sick. My instructor says that I may be able to test for black belt next year, when I'm 50. I'm hoping to enter the second half of my life with better skills and a better attitude.

I'm helping with the training of other students. It's exciting to help someone else learn to be more self-reliant.

There's a facet of martial arts training that's very appealing for people with chemical sensitivities: the non-dyed costume is nontoxic, and lots of us wear white baggy cotton clothing anyway. This isn't like skiing or scuba diving or something where your costume will make you sick.

The training is also helpful because this disease forces you to learn to defend yourself and the people for whom you are responsible. It forces you to define your boundaries. Nobody else can really take care of you with this disease. Either you're going to do it or you're going to die. Pain is a compelling motivator.

In Marin County I lived in subsidized housing for disabled people after my divorce. I thought I'd done all I could with environmental controls and diet. I was having an okay life for someone in her seventies or eighties, but I was in my early forties. I was feeling pretty old and pretty brittle. I'd gotten resigned to that. My social worker was suggesting in-home care and support services because I was falling a lot. I had a real close look at the end of driving and taking care of myself. That was alarming, but I didn't know there was an alternative. I didn't know I had it in me to get as strong as I am now, physically or spiritually.

My move to Arizona was not the result of extensive research or planning. I had become phone friends with Bruce, a person here in Snowflake who has severe neurologic problems and seizures from

MCS. At one point he said, "If you're ever between projects, why don't you come down and see how you do in Arizona?" Finally, when I'd just completed one of the several hundred failures I experienced in the Bay Area with advocacy projects, I decided, heck, I might as well die there as here. I got in the car and just started driving. I didn't realize how far it was to Arizona, let alone to this place. I didn't know how hard it would be to make that drive, or I never would have tried it. When I got here I couldn't walk. I couldn't even get out of my car. Bruce came out and picked me up and took me in the house.

After I was here a few days I was still staggering around, but, with a little help, I was taking care of myself. Gradually I got stronger and we went for a couple of short walks. Bruce said, "What if you don't have to wind up in a nursing home by next year? What if there's an alternative? You can rent a room from me, come back and see what you can do. We'll hook up a phone line for you so you can keep doing your work." I wound up renting rooms from him for two years.

When I first came here I was afraid to give up my apartment in the Bay Area and went back several times. But I had stamina and resilience here that just weren't available in the Bay Area because of the pollution. After I was out here a while we folded up my wheelchair. And, after being oxygen-dependent for years while driving anywhere in California, I never refilled my prescription after moving here to this desert.

After getting settled here I started working on disability-related issues in Arizona. And, interacting with Bruce helped me realize that I had been so focused on trying to change the United States that I hadn't dealt with the fear and pain and fury I carry around. So I got into a counseling program and started taking tae kwon do classes.

I worried that Bruce would get tired of having me underfoot all the time. I make a lot of racket, and the phone rings a lot. I'm a handful to live with, and he needs quiet. Eventually, when he couldn't take it another minute I went to live in the garage of another MCS family, and was very much in danger of losing confidence again and becoming homeless. But people pitched in and helped. Bruce sold twenty acres of his property to my dad for a dollar. My mom and dad chipped in money, and the neighbors chipped in money and labor to build this house. It's a little, sturdy, clean house and it's very, very beautiful.

There are nine households of chemically ill people in this area, so far. Some of the people have had horrible losses, and it's hard not to take that out on each other sometimes. At least we know where it's coming from. Some of the people don't like each other, but we're stuck with each other, just like if we had gone on some really long wagon train journey and got trapped together in this remote place. Even if we get absolutely sick to death of each other, we look out for each other. We have to. Bruce and I talk every day, and the neighbors all touch base often to try to keep each others' morale up, or we would get too lonely and too homesick.

Out here we don't have to worry about whether or not a person is going to spray the rosebushes, polish their fingernails, use hair spray or lawn spray, or get a permanent. We don't have to worry about whether somebody's going to idle their engine all afternoon.

I do my advocacy work right here on the bed, with this phone and Rolodex. I spend too much time on the phone. I have a wonderful dog now, and we spend all our time together. I have a vegetable garden. And now I have a computer from the Department of Rehabilitation here in Arizona so I can try to develop job skills I can do from home—laying out newsletters, writing, and things like that. Learning to defend ourselves, that feels critical to me.

When a person with MCS is subjected to ongoing chemical exposures by the people they live with or near—like in an apartment complex or in their own home—that person is being subjected to domestic assault, to the degree that the exposures are intentional or negligent. It's very demeaning and it undermines the confidence of the person with chemical sensitivities in a way that's very similar to what happens to victims of conventional domestic abuse. The insults and blows happen to people with chemical sensitivities and environmental illness on a daily basis, sometimes on an hourly basis.

When someone calls me for help, I try to figure out where they are and what kind of resources they have. If they've been foiled in a room for twenty years on oxygen, we're going to approach the situation differently than if they have more flexibility and resources. I'll find out what programs in their community offer help to people, because the caller may qualify for services even if the service provider doesn't quite know how to deliver them. We figure out if there's someone near them who might know the ropes, like a doctor who understands, a minister, someone with a porch where you can spend the night, or a battered women's shelter. We'll figure out if there are any warm spots in their environment at all, where it looks like there's some hope of help. There's always hope, although sometimes I can't tell what it is we're hoping for.

It terrifies and angers me that we still don't have safe campgrounds or places to stay for the hundreds of refugees who are on the road right now in the Southwest in search of safe air. Some of these folks are desperate. Some of them are going to live and die in their cars. It is impossible for this to go on without a voice, a loud voice.

Those of us who are strong enough, we are not supposed to be quiet and go away and die. We're not supposed to commit suicide. We have the obligation to say what we see, to share our observations. We're supposed to find one another, to work together, to have some sort of impact on the way our society is organized, and the way the economy impacts life and health. I don't know what else to do. I don't have a better plan.

There's a Bible verse, Proverbs 3:5–6: "Trust in the Lord with all your heart, and do not rely on your own insight. In all your ways acknowledge him, and he will make straight your paths." That's the one we go with.

Southern Stories

Story lends narrative structure to events that might otherwise seem random and meaningless.—Allison Cox and David Albert, the Healing Heart Project

Diane Hamilton
Baton Rouge, Louisiana

Soft-spoken and quietly centered, Diane Hamilton, a former research chemist, has lived with MCS for nineteen years. She is now a teacher of Bible Study Fellowship leaders and the facilitator of a Human Ecology Action League (HEAL) MCS support group. She was a healthy child with no allergies except for a sensitivity to beef at the age of five. A bright student, she skipped her senior year of high school to begin college. From designing a home specifically to meet her environmental needs, to traveling great distances for alternative treatments, Diane has remained vigilant in her pursuit of wellness. Today, her spiritual and physical quests are merging in healing ways she never expected. It was my privilege to be a guest in her Baton Rouge home—a true oasis—and to witness her story.

It's an illness of losses. It's an isolating illness. Things are taken away, taken away, taken away. You get down to almost nothing. But, it's funny, I can't really say I feel a lot of loss now. Realistically, I do have some limitations because of the sensitivities. And yet, I don't dwell on it. I spend my time doing what is within the confines of what I can do.

I put my life into becoming a research chemist. I got my B.S. and Ph.D. in chemistry at Louisiana State University. I was twenty-eight, twenty-nine, something like that. I felt like, if we were going to have a family, we needed to think about that. And I knew better than to get into a job where I was surrounded by chemicals all day and try to get pregnant. There was enough information out about

103

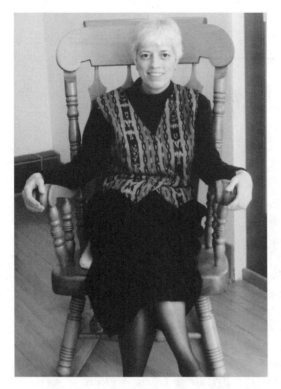

chemicals to know it wasn't wise to do that. So I did post-doc work and delayed getting into a full-time job.

I had difficulty getting pregnant, but within a year I was pregnant. After several months, I was just fatigued. Totally wiped out. I had just enough energy to get up and cook and do things like that. I thought, oh golly, I'm so sick, I'll probably have a sick child. But I had a normal delivery, and my son was very healthy. I was still pretty wiped out after the delivery. I don't know if my body ever recovered, but I gradually got strong and was able to take care of things and enjoyed being a young mother.

We had incredible challenges being new parents, and my husband and I both chose to go into business. He started a software business and I started a specialty chemical business with a former professor. I had loved chemistry labs in college. I loved the investigative part of it. There was some cancer research being done with platinum compounds. We were going to make precious metal chemicals and support research. Later on I realized all the orders we got were for chemicals that were either dangerous, difficult, or deadly.

When my son was two—he's nineteen now—I became sensitive to everything. I had excruciating headaches—almost continual—and sinus congestion, and really hit bottom emotionally.

My grandmother had given me a nutrition book, and it had a section on people who are sensitive. From that book I got a referral to a doctor in Pine Bluff, Arkansas. What I was reading sounded like me, so I thought I'd go and investigate because I wasn't getting anywhere with the doctors here in town. So a friend and I went up there to Arkansas, and that's when I was introduced to chemical sensitivity. He did all kinds of tests, and he said, "You're very chemically sensitive. All these organic solvents that you're around—you can't do that."

I thought, How can I be sensitive to chemicals? I've spent my life preparing for this career! But it was the truth. Every time I would go in the lab I would feel sick; I would get out and I would feel better. But I was still hanging onto my career and business.

I went from place to place trying to get some relief. My husband built a wood structure out on our patio at the house where we lived then. I was desperate, trying to find something that would cure this illness. I lived out on the patio, but if you live outside in Louisiana the mold will get to you. I went across the river, stayed on the back porch of a woman's house while she was in South America for six months; she was the aunt of a friend of mine. And my dear husband—wherever I went it was, "Okay, if you can find some relief here, we'll do it." That's a factor in being able to get to the point where I am, he stood with me. He hasn't fully understood, but he was perceptive enough to know that I wasn't making it up, that what I was going through was real. He never belittled me. That's a big plus, to have someone say, "You need to go across the river to stay on a lady's back porch? Sure, we'll go."

I also stayed at the office building for about six weeks while I was still hanging onto the chemical company. There was an office building and a lab building. Half of the office building was not completed. I stayed there in what was eventually an office, with bare walls, bare floor, a metal bed with cotton blankets. My husband and son stayed there, too. That's the commitment that my husband had.

It is a hopeless feeling you get when you get that isolated. You start thinking is this all there is to life? Is there a God? Why is this happening to me? I started looking at a lot of things. I started reading the Bible again. Previously I'd read bits and pieces, but I started reading it and it started saying things it hadn't said before. It got my attention at that point.

I felt I needed to be getting out of the chemical business we were in. Nobody should be making those kinds of chemicals. But we had invested all this money, all these people had jobs and we had built this building that was specialized. It was an incredible investment.

Then, one day there was an explosion in the lab and a couple of guys got burned. They went to the Baton Rouge burn unit. They recovered, but they could have lost their lives. It really was a jolt. That was a crisis where I got the picture. I thought, God, you don't have to say anything else. That sort of closed the door on that company. It took an explosion for me to quit.

That whole period is still very fuzzy to me. It's hard to remember what happened before the explosion and what happened after. I had such pain in my head and such hopelessness, and that sinking feeling, that I didn't want to go on at one point. How much of my emotional state was related to the trauma at work and how much was part of the chemical sensitivity? I don't think anybody's qualified to answer that.

My husband recognized that he couldn't leave me by myself and he recognized his limitations, so we decided to get some help. I went into a hospital a couple of times. I spent two weeks in a psychiatric unit of a hospital. I needed to separate from what was going on. I wouldn't be here today if I hadn't had some medical intervention. I'm very grateful for that resource. And some good counseling has helped me to express my feelings. But I have battled depression off and on.

There have been different stages in how I have coped with this illness. Very few people have the resources to do what I've done to cope. My home is a safe, quiet haven, and that's had a lot to do with my being able to cope. This place doesn't have gas to it, and I'm very careful about what anybody sprays around here. I've been able to control much of what goes on, and that has helped me.

One important lesson I've learned is to express my feelings. This has been a pivotal lesson for me: When the feelings come, feel the feelings. How long has it taken me to learn this? I'm almost fifty and I'm just getting to the point that I know the importance of expressing my feelings. I'm being relieved. My tongue is being freed. My body is being freed. I'm in the process of being freed.

Keeping a journal has been helpful; I used to write down everything I ate and everything I breathed. And music is a big part. Music speaks to my soul. One of the things I've wanted to do forever is play the piano. I started lessons in July, and that has been another rewarding experience. It's another form of expression.

I've really struggled with being different. Being chemically sensitive is kind of the epitome of being different. It used to bother me. Now, I think I have a healthier view, an acceptance of being different. I'm sure that strikes a familiar chord in anyone who goes through this.

For a while I couldn't be around people because of what they might have on their clothes. I couldn't go to church every week, so I lost that support. My true friends stuck with me and understood, to a point. But I just didn't see people as much, so there were changes in relationships. Others went on with their lives.

I think I have a pretty good perspective on the loss of the chemical career. There are still feelings about that, and yet I don't think too much about wishing I were in a research lab. I really don't, because what I am doing now—teaching for an international, inter-denominational Bible study program—is incredibly fulfilling. It's been a rewarding, challenging process. I'm accepting that I'm called to a different path.

I started participating in the Bible Study Fellowship about thirteen years ago. I was asked to be a children's leader. I did it, enjoyed it, and actually got into a children's supervisory role and was in charge of about a dozen leaders leading about a hundred children, until about four years ago. Then I was asked to teach the leaders for the evening class. I thought, I've never lectured! And I didn't see myself doing that. And yet I felt called to do it. That's what I'm doing now. I have about twenty-two leaders, mostly working women. We meet on Friday mornings. I get up at three-thirty, and we meet from five o'clock in the morning until seven. And then we have classes in the evening. The class has grown from about seventy-five to about a hundred and fifty.

Every time I've gone to another level of leadership there has been a deepening of my spirituality. This study moved beyond religion to getting to know God. More than just going and hearing someone talk about a lesson, this is personal.

I really can say I don't regret what I've gone through, because it's made me what I am. I've thought, God, if you had to pick an illness to show your power, this is as good a scenario as it gets! It drove me to God. The desperation of it forced me to get back to God. I didn't have anywhere else to go. If it took all that I went through to build this testimony, I'm content with that.

All through these years I've continued to look for treatments for the chemical sensitivities. I'm a researcher at heart. I'd keep reading and listening to what was going on. If somebody had a therapy, I'd try it if I thought it was reasonable and wouldn't hurt me. You name a therapy and I've probably done it, I was that intent. Nobody can accuse me of not trying to get well. For a year and a half, every two months I would drive an hour and a half to the airport in New

Orleans, fly to Atlanta, take a subway and taxi to my doctor's office, get a treatment, and return home the same day, wearing a mask the whole way. I'd leave here at six in the morning and get home at nine at night. It was difficult.

Finally I got to the point of wondering, Am I trying too hard? Am I overdoing this search? So I backed off. That was about a year ago.

That fall, a friend sent me a set of tapes made by a minister. I had had it with tapes, and I'd heard people talk about religious healings and I wasn't so sure about that. Then one day during Christmas break I listened to one of them while I was cleaning out a drawer. As I listened I stood there crying. I don't know that I've ever had a response like that to a tape. I think God used this man to reveal something that would take me to the next level of my healing. And it has. I'm in the process of being healed. The minister had some good things to say, but he is not the one who's doing the healing.

I am still chemically sensitive, and just about any food bothers me to some degree. But I'm getting better.

Do I think it's possible to cure my chemical sensitivities? I do! I think it's on its way. I've seen bits and pieces of it already. Fear has been displaced by hope. It's exciting!

Irene Wilkenfeld
Lafayette, Louisiana

While arranging to meet with Diane Hamilton in Baton Rouge, she urged me to include her friend Irene Wilkenfeld. For me, it was a stroke of luck. I had no idea that they were friends or that Irene even lived in Louisiana. I was, however, familiar with her Safe Schools workshops, and certain she would possess a myriad of coping strategies. I was delighted when she agreed to meet me in Baton Rouge for an interview, and disappointed when poor driving conditions prevented her from keeping our appointment. Although I never have met her in person, I experienced her effervescent spirit when we spent

*an evening together by telephone. She has since moved to Cheyenne,
Wyoming, where her husband is now employed.*

*Articulate, bright, determined, energetic, Irene is a delightful
fountain of insight, wisdom and knowledge. Winner of a Most Prom-
ising Foreign Language Teacher Award from Brooklyn College, her
dream career ended in her fifth year of teaching because of MCS.
In a new school with a pesticide-treated foundation, new carpeting
and windows that didn't open, she became completely debilitated
within three months. Fifteen years later her condition was properly
diagnosed. Today she is known for her pioneering work on the sick
school syndrome, and the Safe Schools workshops she presents
across the country.*

———————————

The loss of my teaching career was very major. I had a very distinct loss of self-esteem, I can tell you. I saw myself first as a teacher
and then as a wife and mother. I didn't understand why this person
who had been a lifelong ham suddenly could not be around people.
Every time I went to a movie or any event where there were a lot
of people, I would get very panicky and just want to bolt. People
thought it was agoraphobia. I now know it was because of the fragrances.

Looking back on it, I was a classic case. Chronic bladder infections, panic attacks, gastrointestinal problems, brain fog, weakness,
skin rashes. I was a mass of panic and fatigue. I went to every 'olo-
gist and specialist that there was. None of them was taking a holistic approach. I don't remember any of them ever doing any kind
of occupational or environmental assessment, and it never occurred
to me. I was just as puzzled as puzzled could be. I'm embarrassed to
say it took me fifteen years to find the cause.

Those fifteen years were very hard. I didn't have anyone I could
really talk to and have them understand. I went for counseling during that time, to a psychiatrist for a short while and later to a social
worker. They were lovely people but they had no appreciation of
environmental illness. Whenever something happened that puzzled
me, they would always come up with what seemed like a plausible
reason. Now when I look back I know how foolish they were. For
example, I remember coming away from one session feeling really
good. It was a nice spring day and I drove home with the car

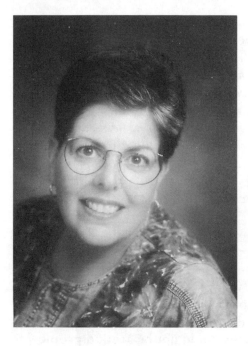

windows rolled down. I started to feel panicky and didn't know what it was. I forced myself to go to the dry cleaners to pick up some clothes. By the time I got home I was just this mass of Jell-O. My kneecaps were jumping and I was trembling and shaking. I called the therapist and told her, and her evaluation was that I must have repressed something really important during the session. Now I know that it was the fumes from the car exhaust and the dry cleaning.

It was a very difficult time. I felt isolated and didn't want to talk about "it" because I didn't know what "it" was. I went from doctor to doctor, hoping I would find an answer. I was tested for rheumatoid arthritis because I was having some serious joint problems. I was tested for lupus. Everything, of course, came back negative. After thousands of dollars' worth of tests and lots of time and energy with this rheumatologist, his diagnosis was that I must have a bowling injury—and I was not a bowler! For me, that was the most comical one. If we can laugh at this illness, that's very therapeutic!

Throughout that whole period of fifteen years when we were so confused and bewildered about what had caused this horrific change in me, my husband always said, "I know it's not in your head, I know it's real, and I know that, ultimately, we will find an answer." So I always had his support. But I had a lot of friends who bailed. My birth family never understood about environmental illness. They still don't. Two of my brother's children are mainstream physicians, graduates of Harvard Medical School, and they think I'm a kook.

About three years after I stopped teaching I met a woman who was writing children's fiction stories. I decided to write and asked her to critique my first little story, called *Mitch and the Little Red Wagon*. She thought it was great, and I sold it for a total of seven dollars and fifty cents. Therein started my writing career. That's what

I did for all those years before I started my sick school syndrome consulting business. I wound up doing a lot of writing about nutrition and food. That kind of laid the groundwork because then I had the facility for writing when I learned about environmental illness and sick building syndrome and sick school syndrome.

I eventually moved to Baton Rouge, Louisiana. I was still very perplexed. I picked up the local paper and in it was a letter written to the editor by someone in the Louisiana chapter of HEAL. It described me. It looked like someone had written my medical profile. There was information on how to contact Diane Hamilton, the leader of the group. I called her the very next day and she arranged to see me that day. I spoke with her at length and she sent me home with a stack of books and articles. I often tease her about how she's changed my life.

Shortly thereafter I called to make an appointment with an environmental physician in Mobile, Alabama, the closest environmental physician to Baton Rouge at that time. I was told I could not be seen until I completed a very extensive patient history form which they would mail to me, and they wanted a picture of me. After I completed that history I started making connections for the first time.

When I arrived for my appointment there was a big red stop sign indicating that you could not enter if you were scented in any way. At that moment I knew that I had found mecca, because one of the hallmarks of my experience, after I became sensitized to formaldehyde and pesticides, was that I suddenly found myself very, very sensitive to perfumes. When I saw that the doctor understood the hazards related to fragrances, I knew I had come to the right place.

Once I found out what it was, I became very active in the Louisiana HEAL organization, so I had an enormous amount of support. That's one of the things that I think is key in this whole issue, really networking. Even though I'm new to Lafayette and don't have a lot of people around me here, I have many supportive friends now all around the country.

I wish I could say it has been a steady climb to health. But actually, it's been cyclical. Since that initial injury I have had two more massive exposures.

I made major improvements under this doctor's care. So much so that two and a half years later, when we were moving to Indiana, I really thought I could develop a new persona in Indiana, that I was healed and could live a normal life.

By this time I thought of myself as something of an "expert"—which I can now laugh about. I had published a couple of articles on safe home construction, and we were having a home built. I gave tons of information to the gentleman who we had contracted with to build our house. We paid extra for alternative construction materials. My husband had really indulged me. We had ordered special ceramic tiles from Germany, and they were just gorgeous.

There was no one on site to supervise the construction process, and it turned out the contractor was less than scrupulous. He used traditional construction materials laden with formaldehyde. My dream house was a nightmare, a toxic soup I had to live in for ten months until we made the contractor buy it back from us.

At that point I got very sick again. Some of the symptoms were the same, many of them were different. My major problem at that point was hives, or eczema, I developed over virtually my entire body, with intense itching that wouldn't stop. I couldn't sleep. I couldn't eat. We had put all of our money into that house. I was a mess. I knew no one there.

At that point I went to meet with a doctor who was doing some interesting work in South Carolina with formaldehyde-sensitive patients. That turned out to be a wonderful experience. I eventually healed from that exposure and was doing really well.

I had no support system there, so I started a HEAL chapter. What happened was, I started to get phone calls from people complaining about conditions in their children's schools. I thought maybe this was an area I needed to look into, so I started doing research. Nobody seemed to have any research on sick schools, so I just started collecting case histories from these parents and, eventually, from teachers who felt the school environment compromised their health. And gradually I started finding bits and pieces about the connection between environmental exposure and brain function—short-term memory loss, the ability to access, store and retrieve information, all of that kind of neurobiology as it related to the environment.

I have collected more than twenty-eight hundred case histories from across the country. You would be appalled at the kinds of situations these youngsters are expected to learn in. If someone is gasping for breath because they're having an asthmatic attack triggered by a classmate's perfume or by a harsh cleaning chemical, there's no way that youngster is going to be able to concentrate on the lesson at hand, even if he has the Teacher of the Year standing in front of him. We're using pesticides prophylactically in the schools and on the campuses—known neurotoxic agents. Classrooms are reeking with mold. Why would intelligent people knowingly expose youngsters in the place where we're supposed to be nurturing brains? They don't get it. I don't know how many times a day I say that to myself, they just don't get it!

Our best educational efforts will be sabotaged unless we really take a look at our classrooms and campus environments. We've read about the increases in asthma in schoolchildren—stunning increases in morbidity and mortality. Recently I came across a statistic, which I think is conservative, that said 12 percent of public school children are classified as medically fragile—meaning they have some major chronic condition such as spina bifida, asthma, heart condition, or they're being treated for leukemia or something of that nature. We're putting these children in classrooms that are reeking with chemical toxins!

Parents are afraid that if they speak out their children will suffer the consequences with bad grades or whatever, and it often happens. Teachers abdicate their power because they're afraid of reprisals or losing their jobs, or being ostracized by some of their colleagues. It will take a process of education. Educators need to be shown medical reports, statistics, and just how environmental exposures in the classroom can affect mood and behavior, academic performance, and students' and teachers' health.

There is a growing awareness of the needs of children. In 1987 I couldn't get any information about the environment and schools from any agency or association. Now I have books and books and books. There's the *Healthy School Handbook*, Dr. Rapp's books, books about preconception care, superimmunity and all kinds of topics. Recently I was contacted by the Agency for Toxic Substances and Disease Registry; they're beginning to establish guidelines to safeguard children. Up in Canada they have a group of pioneering schools in the Kitchener-Waterloo system, with ecoclassrooms. These are environmentally controlled classrooms where they've done everything imaginable to make accommodations for chemically sensitive students and teachers. It's wonderful.

In March of 1988 I did my first workshop on the subject. Very naïvely, because I didn't realize the extent of what I was taking on, I announced that I was going to do a workshop on the sick school syndrome for our support group and community. That's what started it for me. Once the word went out that this was something I was looking at, I started getting calls from all over the United States, Canada, Australia and everyplace. It's just blossomed since then.

A year ago we moved back to Louisiana. I was well enough to travel, and my career with the sick school program really took off. I presented workshops in Canada, Nebraska, several locations in Illinois and Michigan, Faribaut and Bloomington, Minnesota. I was scheduled to be in Duluth in April, but I had to cancel due to my third massive exposure.

I had gone to my first appointment with a doctor in this area, because I had not yet established a relationship with a doctor in Louisiana. I sat in the waiting room very intensely filling out the patient history forms, until I heard what sounded like torrential rain. Within ten seconds I realized it wasn't water, it was pesticides. It turned out to be Dursban TC for termite control. They literally washed the outside of the building with it. There were puddles everywhere. As luck would have it, I was there on the day of this gross misapplication. I have filed a claim with the Department of Agriculture. Ultimately, the pest control company was fined at an adjudicating hearing, and the applicator lost his license for termite treatments in Louisiana. Still, I am troubled because here in this beautiful place the hazards of pesticides are grossly unrecognized.

I suspended my workshops until I recovered from that exposure. Fortunately, I have been able to resume my schedule.

There are times when I'm very angry. What I've found to work for me is, I do all of my venting in the privacy of my home, usually with my husband or over the phone with my daughter. I do it under controlled circumstances because I don't want the outside world to view me as one of those "crazy EIs." I work very hard at being professional and in control when I'm out in public. Like that commercial, "Don't let them see you sweat!" I often use that advice. No one has ever seen the kind of anger that I sometimes feel, with school administrators who don't understand or the mainstream medical community, for example. I'll sometimes emote in the shower. Whatever it takes, but not in front of them.

A field investigator from the Department of Agriculture came to my house two weeks after I filed the complaint about the pesticide misapplication. I was still quite ill, and my first reaction was to tell him what I really thought: How I think they treat the state like a toilet bowl, always cleaning up spills and accidents rather than finding ways to prevent the barge accidents and the explosions and the spills. I really wanted to tell him what I thought about their being in the pocket of all the pesticide manufacturers. I did none of the above. I was very controlled. I had put together a twelve-page chronology of my exposure and the subsequent symptoms I was suffering, information about the company that manufactures Dursban TC and the health hazards associated with exposure to organophosphates. So I got all of that information on the record.

I channel my anger into action. It's one of the ways I cope—and now it's become my modus operandi. I'm always like a detective trying to search out information. Information is power. Knowledge is power. While I was growing up there were no expectations of me other than to make straight As, win scholarships and become valedictorian. I didn't have to make my bed or learn to cook. The only message I ever got was "Study, study, study." I guess I internalized that message. I'm the happiest reading books and gathering information. I love surfing the Net—it's just my way of living my life.

Those tools are serving me very well with this illness. There are times when I get so excited if I find a new fact or I'm looking for a reference and I locate it. For me it's a challenge. I love doing it.

I am a master of strategies for taking care of myself when I travel. For example, I never plan back-to-back trips. I tend to be a delayed reactor, so I fly to a location the day before my workshop and I fly home the day after it. I'm starting to react by the day after I come home. Before I go and after I'm back I soak in a bath with either baking soda, Epsom salts, apple cider vinegar or hydrogen peroxide. Long hot soaking baths. That really seems to help me detoxify. I take a large protocol of supplements, some specifically for when I fly. I also travel like a gypsy, my husband says, with my own bed linens and my own bath towels. My host or hostess understands my situation better than the average person, so they often run interference for me and are very helpful in helping find me a motel room. It has to be a non-smoking room with a window that opens, in a facility that has not been recently renovated, pesticided or had new carpeting installed. I'm finding, more and more, that people are willing to accommodate a request to clean the room with just water or vinegar or something of that nature. Very often, too, my host or hostess will put a HEPA filter in the room the night before and get things ready for me. Also, while I'm gone I drink only filtered water, I eat light and, as much as possible, organic food.

In order for me to accept an invitation to speak, I make certain requests about the facility where the presentation will be given: no recent pesticide applications, no harsh cleaning products, preferably windows that open and no carpeting. When the announcements go out inviting people to the workshop, they are asked to come unscented.

It has worked surprisingly well for me. If someone wearing a scent approaches me, and the scent is so strong that I feel that I'm going to have Cool Whip on the brain, I tell them "I'm very sorry, I'm certain that the scent you have on is lovely, but it's causing a problem for me. Can you step back or can we talk about this outside in the fresh air?" A lot of people don't realize that, even if their deodorant or some other product says it's unscented, it might have a masking fragrance in it or something of that nature. If it's mild and I don't notice any immediate reaction, I usually don't make a big fuss about it. But see, after I've talked about the neurotoxic effects of perfumes in my workshop, they won't approach me if they know they're scented, if they have any smarts.

More often than not, the people responsible for my coming to a workshop are not the administrators, they are the parents and injured teachers who are going through that loss of self-esteem and feeling that all of their influence has been taken from them. They're feeling isolated and ostracized. I share with them my story and the stories of others who have recovered, to show them that there is life after chemical injury and that no one can take your power away from you unless you allow them to.

What I've found is: this illness is cyclical. You might be in the depths of despair and illness one moment, but then the body does have an uncanny ability to repair itself, if not to recover fully, to at least improve noticeably.

The first thing I say to a person with MCS who is feeling desperate is, "It's not always going to be like this." Each time I've had a massive exposure and gotten sick, I thought that was it, it was going to be chronic and would always be that bad or downhill from there. When this last poisoning occurred, I was devastated. I was quite sick and depressed. I thought, now I've had my second career stolen from me! But that's not the case. I am on the road again, and in the interim I did telephone consultations and research and what have you.

This illness has its peaks and valleys. Sometimes I feel so good that I almost think that I don't have to deal with this anymore. But I always have to be cognizant of the facts, and vigilant, I think, so

I can avoid the next crash. I look beyond the problems to see the challenges or benefits or a door that I can open. I have to be a little bit creative in problem solving. There are alternatives for everything. You don't have to do things in the same way that you've always done them. For example, people say, "I have to use pesticides, I live in Louisiana and we have flying roaches!" Well, I lived in Louisiana for twelve years before we moved, and I have not used pesticides since 1985, and I don't have pests in my house.

We have the gift of intelligence, which should lead to flexibility and looking at what our options really are.

I'm learning to relax with myself and appreciate who I am and know that I don't have to stand on top of the mountain all the time. I used to just kind of steel myself for the fight. I'm really learning to relax more. I exercise every day. I give voice to my feelings and allow myself to cry or be lazy if I'm feeling low, but I don't allow it to become routine. I give myself permission to wallow in my feelings, and then—that's it girl! Get back into gear! I try to be my own best friend.

I love to garden. I love to bike ride. If you can believe it, I rollerblade! My husband and I love sightseeing and nature. I love to read. I don't have a minute that I don't have something I like to do. I'm never bored. And now I am a new grandmother!

Keeping a schedule during the work week is very positive for me. When I'm well I come into my office every morning at nine o'clock. I work, I take a lunch break, I do about forty-five minutes of exercise, I come back into the office. I'm very, very regimented.

If there's one thing that still makes me anxious, it's having to deal with a myopic mainstream health care professional. It's almost like it's imprinted in my body. Those fifteen years when I was searching for answers, I think I was abused, in some instances, by less than caring physicians who didn't understand and who wanted to discard me into their medical wastebaskets because I wasn't good for their ego, because I would have an adverse reaction to whatever prescription they wrote for me. I just didn't fit into their cookie-cutter mold, you know.

Before I go to a doctor I prioritize what is critically important for me to get across to them. Sometimes I role-play before I go, and I establish my boundaries: What am I willing to be flexible about? I have to know when to say, "This won't work for me, I think we'll have to agree to disagree and I will have to look elsewhere."

Awareness of this illness is definitely growing, though. And I hope to continue to play my role in that area.

I don't think anyone would choose this illness. But if this is your lot in life—you know what they say about making lemonade. When I look back over these last bunch of years I think there have been benefits. I've met some extraordinarily bright, intelligent, caring, communicative, insightful people. I've gained a real appreciation for ecology—a word I didn't know the meaning of when I was growing up. I really think that I am now a born-again environmentalist, and I have a whole different perspective on the world. It is not better living through chemistry. Anyone who still believes that if a product is on the market in the United States then it must be safe, needs to go back to school. That's a very naïve attitude. We are degrading the planet by this addictive use of chemicals for every possible situation. Now, I wish I didn't have liver damage, and I wish I didn't have hives, and I wish I didn't itch and all of those things, but I've grown a great deal as a person.

There is definitely an upside.

Linda Angeles
Pensacola, Florida

While working in a school and in the lawn maintenance business, Linda Angeles became severely ill. Although she knew that certain chemical exposures made her sick, she had no idea to what extent. It took her years to understand there was a relationship between chemicals and her chronic illness. In an effort to reclaim her health, she left an unhappy marriage and now lives alone in a trailer.

One of Linda's primary reactions to chemicals is joint and muscle pain so severe that even walking is difficult for her. Another common reaction for her is cognitive impairment. She carries oxygen in her car in case she has a chemical reaction while driving. A significant loss she has experienced due to MCS is access to her church.

Still, her spirit and spirituality prevail. She embraces joy and compassion along with grief and sorrow. Her smile is warm, her laughter joyous. She is a mother and grandmother. And she paints greeting cards and makes other crafts that are absolutely delightful.

———————————

Most people think of me as a hard worker. Part of my caring for people was physically doing things for others. If there was something that needed to be done, I'd do it. One woman once said, "I can't believe it, Linda Angeles is sitting eating her lunch, she's not working!" I guess it was a way of coping.

I was a very, very physically active person. I wouldn't have taken an elevator or walked up stairs, I would have *jumped* up two or three at a time, spontaneous, like a child!

I'd love it if someone said, "Hey, you wanna go to Birmingham?" I'd say, "Yeah, let's go!" But then, because of my sensitivities, my mind would start clicking: Where are you going to sleep? How are you going to sit in the car with fumes? But I still want to do it. I want people to care enough to find out what they can do so that we can enjoy each other's company.

I've been chemically sensitive for a long time, but I did not know what that was. I always knew that when new carpet went into a home or a store, I couldn't go there. I knew I could not tolerate anyone's perfume or to wear it myself. Mold would elicit asthma symptoms. I could not stand the fumes from the chemicals used by exterminators in the school where I worked. I knew that I was very sensitive to certain medications.

Every year there was some major remodeling project at the school where I worked. The fumes even made people who weren't as sensitive as me sick. I liked my job and needed to work, so I'd tell myself "You can make it to Labor Day" and then "You can make it to Thanksgiving." By Christmas it would be affecting me so badly that I could hardly cope physically or emotionally. Then I still had to make it through the rest of the year. I was doing landscaping and yard grooming three-quarters of the year, so I was working two, sometimes three jobs.

In 1989 I had pneumonia and I have never been well since. I know, now, that is where I crossed the line with chronic fatigue and chemical sensitivity.

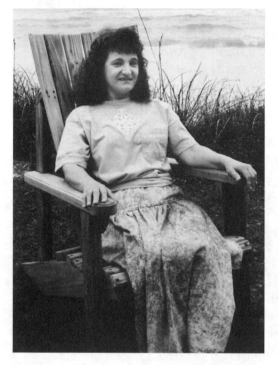

I knew I had to leave my marriage in order to take care of myself. So I purchased a little travel trailer to live in. I had no electricity, no toilet facilities, but I had peace and quiet.

Two years later I bought a stationary trailer, like a small mobile home. I thought that if I bought a new trailer I wouldn't have mold problems; I didn't think about the formaldehyde and what it would do to my health. Even though I bought two fans and put them in the windows to pull the air out, I had bronchitis really bad by that evening. I had to disconnect the gas stove and central heat. I cook on a hot plate, which isn't much fun.

When I am exposed to chemicals I drift around. It takes me a long time to realize what is going on, and I lose sight of how much time has gone by. I'll look at everything in a store, and be simply amazed that it's gotten dark outside. There's nobody to tap me on the shoulder and say, "You need to go outside and change the air," or, "You need to go lay down in your car," or "You need to go eat."

There are times when it is not safe for me to get behind a wheel, because my reactions are slowed from exposures to chemicals. Once I was in a car accident because an elderly man ran a stop sign. I saw that he wasn't stopping, but my mind was so slow from a chemical reaction that I couldn't respond in time, and he caught the tail end of my car. So there was more pain and more inactivity. It became a cycle. I couldn't go back to work and I was losing everything. I had no strength, the pain was horrible. I thought the pain was caused by the car accident, but nobody could tell me what was wrong.

At one point I was hospitalized for depression. They kept pouring medicine into me and it made everything horribly worse. I couldn't think, I couldn't smile, my landlady said my conversation made no sense. Right in the middle of a sentence I would change the subject, and I didn't think anything was wrong. That's what medications and other chemicals can do to me, even antibiotics. When I tell doctors the side effect, they don't believe me. Not being believed is the hardest part, and knowing they think I'm a hypochondriac or crazy.

It was three years before I found out I was reacting to chemical exposures. When I was tested, one of my reactions to chemicals was an inability to move or respond. By then my physical condition had also deteriorated from inactivity.

I'm one of Jehovah's Witnesses, and even that has suffered from my chemical sensitivities. I would go to the Kingdom Hall for Bible study and have to lie on the floor, I was so weak and close to passing out. People would say, "Did you have a good sleep?" And I would say, "I wasn't sleeping. If you looked at me and observed me you would think I was, but I hear everything you're saying, I just cannot move or respond to you."

Several years ago I realized I could no longer go into the Kingdom Hall. I do have a telephone hookup now. I can listen but I can't participate, so that is another isolation. Last night I gave a talk. I had to tape it, and the tape was played in the hall. It was exciting for me, but I cried because the normal thing would be for me to be there with my brothers and sisters.

We have conventions or assemblies three times a year. I have two children who are in the same religion, but I drive myself to the conventions and stay alone in the motel because my children will have fresh perm in their hair, or cologne, or dry-cleaned clothes. At the auditorium, where there are thousands of people, I am horrendously sick. But I can't give that up, too. I've already given up the three weekly meetings because I just can't expose my immune system to that much. I know I'm going to be sick wherever I go, it's just a matter of degree and how alert I'm going to be. It's made my life completely different, everybody who knows me can tell you that.

I got to the point where I couldn't vacuum or stand and cook for myself. I've gotten better since I've been treated for some of the chemical sensitivities and some of the allergies to relieve the stress on my immune system. But I can't go into stores or malls—it's become very dangerous for me—and I don't have a social life, except for a couple of friends I'm in contact with. At this time in my life I should be able to visit friends in other places, but I cringe at traveling because where am I going to stay? And how am I going to function? Even accepting an invitation to go to lunch is hard because I don't know if there will be people wearing dry-cleaned clothes or perfume. I'm also afraid if I keep saying no because I'm not feeling well, I'll never be invited again. I'm kind of isolated.

I need hugs, and now I don't want them anymore because it's not safe. In order to see my grandchildren I pay dearly. I have to ask myself, how sick do you want to be and how many days can you afford to be down? I don't know how to *be* anymore. MCS has stunted my emotional growth.

Sometimes I cry for the sadness of what I've lost. It's like there's a river trying to get over the mountain and come down. I remember once, after a flood of tears, when I went outside the trees were so green and I could breathe and I could talk to Jehovah again. I remember that same feeling another time, after I cried and cried, when afterwards the colors of the buildings and the sky and trees were so beautiful and clear.

My spiritual hope is what keeps me going. Jesus was not a wimp, and he expects me to be bold and courageous in sharing my spiritual hope. To help me do that, I have only to ask God and He will give me power beyond what is normal for me. That's in the scripture. I have a great worldwide family in the congregation, wherever I may go in the world, and that's a good feeling.

I've come a long way. I can walk now, even though it takes me a while. I'm more aware of everything in life, extremely aware of the environment. I've given myself permission to feel and do things that I wouldn't before. MCS has slowed me down to the point where I've had to face up to me and be with me. It has cut down on my "running," which is how I coped since I can remember. I'm much more understanding and tolerant and patient, to my imperfect degree. I can tell others that it's okay to feel angry, that even Jehovah God expressed anger, and David was very expressive of his feelings. It's okay to feel your feelings.

I sometimes give myself permission to have knock-down-drag-out major depressive episodes, with suicidal thoughts and everything, because that's how sad I feel, or how hurt. But I would not take my life. I can't disappoint Jehovah, and I could not do that to my family or friends. I know the depression will pass.

It really helps me to have a structured routine, to have a schedule similar to when I worked. I used to make a written schedule. I feel useful when I check something off, I feel I've accomplished something. My goal is to spend quality time bonding with and making memories for my grandchildren to cherish.

One of the things I've learned is to have fun, and I've learned to have a better sense of humor. I've always had a sense of humor but I didn't show it off. The first time I said something that made people laugh, it was like Valium. I got on a roll and just kept going. I often laugh and make fun of the things I do or my illness. I use it as a coping mechanism, and it helps other people to be able to talk and relax. Humor is a big part of me now.

What is most important to me now is to be able to make a difference, spiritually, with other people, to tell them not to be afraid to reach out, and to know that the Bible was written for our benefit, in our current lives. Even if they don't want to study the Bible or do anything about their spiritual life, I can lead them to tools to give them hope.

I haven't given up hope of participating in activities I used to enjoy. I never would throw away my ice skates, even though my kids always said, "Nobody's gonna have an ice skating rink in Pensacola!" I said, "One day, somebody's gonna build me one," and they did! I don't know if I can physically put on the skates and skate now, but one day I'm gonna ask somebody to sharpen my skates, and somebody to hold my hand, and do it!

California Stories

New paradigms are nearly always received with coolness, even mockery and hostility. Their discoveries are attacked for their heresy... But the new paradigm gains ascendance... When a critical number of thinkers has accepted the new idea, a collective paradigm shift has occurred.—From *The Aquarian Conspiracy* by Marilyn Ferguson

Carolyn Martin
Emeryville, California

It is easy to picture Carolyn Martin in the roles she enjoyed before her chemical injury: patron of the arts, museum docent, symphony season-ticket holder, political fundraiser, socialite and traveler, to name a few. Beautiful clothes and home furnishings gave her pleasure in her former life. Now her wardrobe consists of several pieces of safe clothing, and a large collection of beautiful scarves used to soften the blow of chemical exposures. Draped strategically over her shoulder, she will pull a scarf up to cover her nose and mouth when a waft of fragrance or other chemicals hits her out in public.

In the few hours I spent with Carolyn, I was blessed by her humor, sadness, dignity, humility, inspiration and grace. My brief encounter with her illustrates some of the seriousness and the subtleties of MCS, and the frustration of people with this illness—and those who interact with them—when extensive planning and precautions still end with spoiled plans.

Carolyn, fifty-four when interviewed, is confined to a wheelchair because of multiple sclerosis, diagnosed in 1980. After the onset of MS she continued to enjoy her status as a fiercely independent woman until a chemical injury changed her life in 1989. Now, because her reactions to chemical exposures can be life threatening, she is dependent upon personal attendants twenty-four hours a day. Upon first meeting Carolyn I had no idea her reactions were so serious, nor did I realize she frequently had to be rushed to a hospital emergency room to save her life. Our meeting came dangerously close to ending in tragedy, although I didn't realize it at the time.

Carolyn had insisted on coming, with her driver, to pick me up where I was staying in San Francisco to bring me to the high-rise where she lives in the East Bay for the interview. She was afraid that if I took public transportation I would be exposed to so many chemicals on the way that I wouldn't be in any shape to really hear and understand what she had to say. What I didn't know was that riding into the city was a terrific challenge for her, and that she was protecting me at the expense of her own health.

Upon arrival at her residence her driver lifted her out of the car and into an electric chair. Then Carolyn dismissed her attendant for the duration of the interview. Instead of going to her apartment, we went to a quiet public room in the building, because she thought some work being done in her apartment would be distracting. Before I had even set up my recorder, Carolyn calmly told me that she was having a reaction to something in the room. To me it looked like she was simply yawning in an odd, repetitive sort of way, and I continued setting up for the interview. When I pulled out some papers, her reaction worsened. Unsure what do to, I asked for her direction. In a tiny whisper she croaked out that she needed to get outside. So I packed up my things and followed her in what felt like a kind of daze. It never occurred to me that her throat was closing and I should drop everything and rush her out the door in her wheelchair. It was a typical and terrifying scenario for Carolyn, to have the people around her underestimate the seriousness of the situation. Her attendant, who would have known what to do, was not around, and Carolyn was thinking "the end was near." Fortunately, outside in the fresh air she managed to take the medication that can save her life.

In retrospect, I was stunned by my failure to act appropriately in the moment. Part of the reason was because I had lost sight of the fact that chemical reactions can be fatal, and because Carolyn's reaction was, for the most part, invisible. I also did not understand how dependent she was on her attendants in these kinds of situations. However, another major factor was that I'd been exposed to the smell of fragrances, dryer sheets and cleaning products that morning in the bed and breakfast where I was staying. My exposure had been brief and I thought I was recovered, but in fact my thinking and reactions were still considerably dulled. This was a wake-up call.

Still determined to make a contribution to this book, Carolyn made another attempt—this time outside—to do the interview after her medication had started to take effect. Afraid that her soft voice would be carried away by the breeze, I tried to attach the tape recorder to the handlebars of her chair, as close to her mouth as possible. As I stood smack dab in front of her chair trying to secure the recorder, she really got excited and began to croak, "Take it off! Take it off!" Inadvertently I had placed the tape recorder on her hand-operated accelerator! After that episode we laughed hysterically for a few moments, imagining how it might have looked if an out-of-control electric chair had mowed me down and carried Carolyn off to her demise.

Believe it or not, we made several more attempts to have the interview. Just when we thought we were finally situated, the smell of pesticides drifted our way and we had to make another move. Finally, Carolyn had the presence of mind to realize that the interview should be discontinued because she was so ill and so exhausted from the whole ordeal. Extremely disappointed and feeling that she had somehow failed, she apologized profusely.

Her voice is soft and smooth as silk, barely audible at times as a result of chemical exposures. In addition to chemicals she is extremely sensitive to light and sound, including the sound of her own voice. When I asked her to speak a little more loudly to ensure that her voice would be recorded on tape, she responded incredulously with, "You mean I'm not shouting?" Her eyes are beautiful reflecting pools often hidden behind dark glasses, because her eyes turn blood red and burn when exposed to bright light.

Carolyn is the mother of one child, a grown daughter.

People understand what they can see. You cannot see MCS. My reactions look like an anxiety attack, so people think "Oh, she's having an anxiety attack." They don't respond to the situation for what it is, because they don't understand.

Fortunately, my doctor is very understanding. Once, when my throat was closing and my eyes were swelled, my daughter called him and he said, "Does she have prednisone?" My daughter said, "Yes, but they've expired. Can't we just go to the hospital?" He said, "She won't make it to the hospital! Give them to her now!"

It's terrifying to go out with someone, wondering if they will understand and act appropriately if I have a chemical reaction. I'm

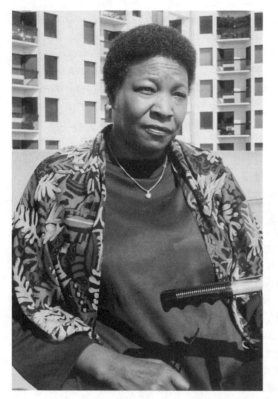

apprehensive about making new friends because of the time and effort it takes to make them aware of what happens to me, so that I can survive if I'm exposed to chemicals when we're out together. Now, I spend most of my time with my attendants who are trained to respond instantly.

Many of my old friends—who were sensitive to my needs when I was confined to a wheelchair—have fallen by the wayside because they couldn't understand my need for them to refrain from wearing fragrances. Some wrote me off as a mental case.

The people who live here in my building are very understanding, because they've seen me rushed away in an ambulance time and time again. They'll inform me of any work being done on my floor, and will take me out the back door if there's something toxic in the lobby.

My daughter is very understanding. Thankfully, so are the people who work in the emergency room at the hospital. At one point I was winding up in the ER almost every other night. My attendant always checks out the ambulance first, to make sure there's nothing in there that will finish me off when I get in. Being dependent upon other people to make my life work has been the most difficult adjustment for me.

My chemical injury happened when I had my attic insulated in my three-story house in Piedmont. Apparently it wasn't done properly, and the fiberglass and cellulose fell down into my living quarters. Consequently, it contaminated everything in the house.

I was in the habit of filling the house with plants and flowers once a month. One of the first things I noticed after the insulation was installed was that the plants and flowers died. Then I noticed

I wasn't feeling well, but I didn't realize it was from something in the house until I sprained my ankle and had to stay inside. Once I was on bedrest, I began to get very ill. My eyes turned blood red and burned so from exposure to light that I was almost blind and had to wear sunglasses or a blindfold when I went outside. I coughed constantly and my throat sometimes felt like it was closing. My face and body swelled to enormous proportions and I lost control of my bladder.

Prior to this experience I'd never had symptoms of being sensitive to anything. I had never been unusually sick since the day I was born in Louisiana.

Thinking it was something in my bedroom making me ill, I moved to every bedroom in the house to see if I'd get better. But instead, I got progressively worse. This went on for months and months, and I went from doctor to doctor. Many were supportive and offered me diagnoses, everything from lymphoma to lupus. Others asked me, "Have you seen a psychiatrist lately?" Of course, I had none of these problems.

I was being poisoned from the toxins in my environment. I finally started to figure that out after I went to live in a girlfriend's apartment while she was out of town. During that time I started to feel much better, but I didn't improve one hundred percent because I took some of the contaminated goods with me from my house.

Then an allergist came to my house, examined samples of the insulation, and told me that it was poisoning me. By then I was so sensitive that I had to get rid of most of my things, including three closets-full of clothes. Somehow I was put in contact with Susan Molloy, who was involved with a support group in the area, and she said she would get some clothes for me that I could probably tolerate. When I went over to Marin County to get them from her I was wearing an amethyst and diamond ring. Susan took one look at it and said, "I don't know if you'll wear these clothes—look at that ring!" I told her it was one of the few things I wasn't reacting to. And I wore those old used clothes for a long time. Elegance, and all the "things" that once were so important to me, no longer mattered.

Eventually I moved from my eleven-room house to a one-bedroom apartment. My apartment is sparsely furnished. I can't have beautiful furniture or a beautiful sofa because I'm sensitive to many woods and fabrics now. Everything has to be silk or cotton.

My life didn't stop with MS. When I was first diagnosed I

thought, okay, I can't ski and I can't play tennis, but there are many things I *can* do. Then I explored the world of things I still could enjoy, like going to the symphony and art museums. When I lost the use of my legs I replaced them with a wheelchair. MS presented me with a challenge, to create a different world for myself. The world I created was beautiful, really, and I remained very independent.

Now I have to create another world for myself, one with even more limitations. But I still have the ability to replace my losses. For example, I can no longer go to the symphony, but I can purchase tapes. I can't go to many public places but I can still enjoy nature. What is most important to me now are the simple things we take for granted. Like being able to breathe. Waking up. Experiencing a beautiful day. Quite often I ask my attendant to take me for a drive near the ocean, where I can breathe fresh air. This is how you find a new way. This is how you get quality out of life.

Jack Ronan
San Francisco, California

By the time I reached Jack Ronan's office in the Financial District of San Francisco, my nerves were jangled from a crowded bus and chemical exposures. Soon after we settled into a quiet corner of a salad bar restaurant for the interview, Jack's calming spirit had rubbed off on me.

Jack has suffered with what may have been traditional allergies since birth. His breathing was so labored as an infant that his sister could hear him sleeping from another room. His mother recognized his reactions to milk and juice, but put them back into his diet when she thought that he was better. As a child he was constantly tired, his skin itched and he was sensitive to the sun. Despite the fact that he always felt sick and his symptoms persisted all year long, it was assumed that his problem was hay fever. Years later, after cigarette smoking had compounded his problems, he learned that he was reacting to a broad range of foods and environmental triggers.

Jack, fifty-eight when interviewed, studied French at Georgetown University. He currently works in computer programming and is looking forward to a career change or retirement in the near future.

Anybody with MCS is really courageous. We're survivors. Stronger—mentally—than most of us probably realized. It's amazing what we go through. We're all heroes. There's no doubt about that.

I've been unhealthy all of my life but didn't realize I was chemically sensitive until I stopped smoking, in my thirties. Before that I felt so dead tired and sick all the time that I didn't know when I was reacting to chemical exposures. I couldn't understand what was wrong with me. After I quit, when I was around someone smoking a cigarette I felt like someone had stuck a hot poker up my nose. It was extremely painful. Now I have a chronic sinus condition and I am never without pain for one second, and I get sick from exposures to perfume, cleaning products and things like that, and many foods.

I think most people who have MCS don't even know it. Others don't tell anyone for fear that people will either think they're crazy or won't believe them. There is stigma and shame associated with having this illness. There have even been news stories making fun of people who ask others not to wear perfume to meetings.

There needs to be a lot more education so people realize just how serious and widespread MCS is. It's not a funny thing. There needs to be more emotional support groups for people living with this illness.

When I was a kid I thought everybody felt awful all the time. I didn't have a great deal of confidence in myself, because it's hard to feel good about yourself when you feel sick. After I started smoking in college I felt worse than ever. Amazingly enough, I was actually a good student.

When I realized I was reacting to fragrances and other chemicals, I went to see a doctor who discovered that my main problem was food allergies. He told me that my chemical intolerances would improve from eliminating the foods I'm allergic to from my diet. I have found that to be true. Changing my diet has made a big difference for me. I've learned that eating foods I'm allergic to causes me to feel bloated and hungry, and that I will crave the foods that make me sick. When I eat foods that I'm allergic to, my skin—which is always

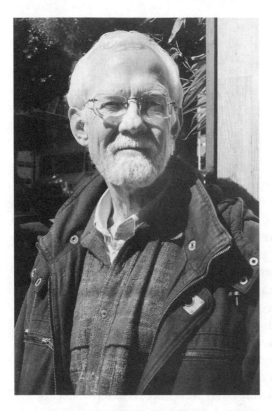

red from sensitivities—gets more inflamed than ever, I feel dead tired and my brain gets real hazy.

The foods I can eat are now very limited. Mostly chicken, fish and vegetables. I cook most of my own meals and almost never eat out in a restaurant except for lunch, and then I eat only salad. I've just learned how to deal with it and I feel so much better that I want to tell people: You don't know how good you'd feel if you stopped eating all those things you really love that aren't good for you! But I don't want to be a proselytizer.

My life hasn't changed a lot since I've identified my food and chemical sensitivities. I still do most of the things I've always done, like go to church and work in an office building. Occasionally I smell things at work that drive me up the wall. When that happens I sometimes take a walk around the block. Whatever was going through the air system is usually cleared up by the time I come back. I had more problems when smoking was allowed in the building. It was impossible to get away from that.

The Unitarian Church that I belong to has designated six fragrance-free pews in one corner for people with chemical sensitivities. People there are very aware of environmental health issues and don't even sit near those pews if they are wearing a fragrance. The choir members have all been supportive too.

The most painful loss I've experienced, partly as a result of my health, was the loss of a twenty-three-year relationship that I thought would last forever. In one of our last counseling sessions together my partner said, "He's running around with people wearing gas masks, for God's sake!" He also told the woman who cleaned our house that she could go back to using a disinfectant on the floors. It was absolutely devastating. I felt disgusted and degraded. It's hard for me to even think about getting involved in another relationship. I spend a lot of time alone now.

Solitude, I've found, can be quite wonderful. Our culture says there's something wrong with you if you want to be alone, but I don't think that way at all. I take my dog for long walks. My mother lives in the area, so I see her. And I do have friends who I see occasionally. But I'm more comfortable being alone now, getting to know myself better. I'm sort of an introvert by nature, and now I've begun to realize that's okay. I certainly get lonely a lot, but I know that's something that will pass and I will be okay. My feelings of loneliness go up and down like everything else. Getting to know myself better and appreciating who I am has helped me through the loss of my partner.

This disease really makes me look at myself and forces me to be more open with others. I think that's really good. Letting people know what is happening to me and facing up to myself have helped a lot.

I need to stay in touch with who I am deep down. The real me. The voice behind the noise. That wonderful silence inside that is a true joy. For me, meditation is the way to get to my joyful spirit. I meditate for twenty minutes twice a day.

When I first started to meditate, thirty years ago, it hurt physically and mentally. That is the very time when it is important to continue. I've had to learn to move through those feelings and to face the emotions inside. I have to pay close attention to thoughts about anger and fear. Beyond those feelings I find a joyful spirit there. I'm really glad I've gone within to find that.

Sometimes it's really hard for me to get past my anger or brain fog or depression or fear. I think part of the depression and self doubt are a result of never feeling well. And part of the reason a lot of people with MCS feel fearful and angry, or depressed, is because this illness works on the part of the brain that controls the emotions.

People usually see me as a mild-mannered person, but there are times when I react to exposures with anger and rage. It's a chemical reaction. I try to get it out in the privacy of my home. My dog Murphy is the only one who hears me vent my anger, and he's pretty used to it now!

When I feel angry I sometimes blame myself for this illness because I used to smoke. But I try to think about it rationally so that

I won't take it out on myself. I am sick from foods and chemicals, including cigarette smoke. I also try not to blame the people who are wearing products that make me sick, because most people don't realize what they are wearing.

Something else that helps me to feel calm and peaceful is to get away from all the auto emissions and pollution. I drive out into Marin County and sit by a creek.

Sometimes I feel great and I have no idea what I've done to make me feel that way. I want to hang onto that feeling forever. There are good days and bad days, good moments and bad moments. That's the way life is.

In the darker moments I wonder how long I can go around feeling lousy all the time. There have been times when I've wanted to just say good-bye. Although I don't have those kinds of thoughts anymore, I don't think they are unusual during difficult periods in life. A lot of people feel that way at times. I try to recognize that, and to remember that no matter how dark it gets, something good will happen.

Learning to live with the ups and downs has made me a stronger person.

Barbara Wilkie
Berkeley, California

Growing up in St. Louis, Missouri, Barbara Wilkie and her brother both suffered with chronic, severe coughing. She vividly recalls when her mother made the comment that they'd almost "lost" her brother. Barbara wondered how he could possibly be lost when his loud coughing made his presence so obvious.

Barbara's father was a physician who saw patients in an office in their home. She instinctively learned to avoid contact with the patients who wore colognes or smelled of powder. Whenever one of the scented patients came too close to her, it set off a coughing fit and she would lose her voice.

As a teenager Barbara moved to the Ozarks with her family. She pitched hay, cleaned animal pens and worked in the gardens without any ill effects. Feathers and dust produced no traditional allergy symptoms.

In adulthood Barbara made her home in California with her husband and three children, the same home where she currently resides. In 1975 she began working for a regional government agency. During workplace renovations in the 1980s, her health began to deteriorate. About that time, in her forties, she was diagnosed with chemically induced asthma and learned that exposures to chemicals and fragrances were contributing to her decline. After she asked for reasonable accommodations in her workplace, she was ostracized and harassed by coworkers for twelve years, until she retired last year. Those years were extremely painful for her both physically and emotionally, and brought back tears as she told the story.

*In one of her most difficult moments Barbara vowed that when she retired she would devote herself to increasing awareness of environmental health issues to improve conditions for others in similar situations. Today she is keeping her word with a burning passion. She is on the board of directors of the Environmental Health Network (EHN) based in Larkspur, California. She is editor of the EHN newsletter—*New Reactor—*maintains a Web page, and helps to field calls on the EHN support and information hotline. She has worked with San Francisco city officials to develop a sustainable city plan. She was one of the authors of a fragrance-free resolution adopted by the Sierra Club.*

Barbara met me in San Francisco for the interview. By the time she arrived her voice was a raspy whisper because of chemical exposures she encountered on her way. Her story illustrates some of the challenges and chemical barriers faced by many people with MCS in their workplaces.

In the late '70s I started asking for help from my manager in curtailing some of the perfume in the workplace. I only knew it aggravated my asthma, but I still didn't know why. My manager said she'd never heard of fragrances causing problems and wouldn't touch the issue. In the early '80s I was diagnosed with chemically induced asthma.

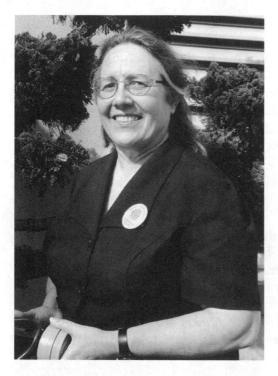

My condition worsened in the mid–'80s when we moved into a newly-renovated building with new carpeting and other finishes, although I still didn't make the connection. I knew the chemical exposures were related to my coughing, but didn't understand the connection to my more serious chronic illness.

An incident in '92 pushed me unmistakably over the cliff into the abyss of MCS. I was at an outdoor ball game with my family when a woman wearing a strong cologne sat down in front of me. I started coughing outrageously and developed an instant sinus infection—as unbelievable as that sounds. By the next morning my ears were so plugged I was totally deaf and in excruciating pain. Medications didn't work and asthma inhalers made me worse. I had laryngitis so bad I didn't know if my voice would ever come back. After five weeks I recovered from that episode, but I felt like I was in a malaise unlike any I'd ever experienced.

Every day it was a struggle to go into my workplace, my reactions to fragrances were so intense. I tried to explain it to people at work, and asked that people call to warn me before coming into my office if they were wearing a fragrance. Many of them were supportive. When they called I'd put on a mask or respirator. But there were some who would walk right in wearing fragrances and get right in my face with no warning, so I'd put on my respirator and continue talking as though nothing was different. One woman told me she was not about to listen to me about fragrances, and she would wear them wherever and whenever she wanted to. It was bad enough to have my peers treat me this way, but even worse was that some of them were managers.

Over time my symptoms worsened and became even more dis-

concerting. Suddenly the right side of my face, from my temple to my
jaw, would become numb, and would stay that way for hours or days.
Or, I'd be walking along engaged in animated conversation, when
suddenly I would feel like the floor or pavement had come up and
hit me in the face, causing me to stumble into a wall, or to black out
momentarily and fall. Twice I fell in front of moving cars. After one
falling episode when I was with my husband, he saw me starting to
go down again and yelled, "Put on your mask!" He detected the scent
of fabric softener in the air, and he made that anecdotal connection.
You've got to play Sherlock to make these connections, but sooner
or later it will click. Once I finally figured out that exposure to fabric softeners made me fall, I've never had the problem again because
I protect myself by putting on my mask at the first hint of it. Even
in my own house I wear a mask when the smell of dryer sheets from
my neighbor's laundry drifts into my house. I've also never had the
numbness in my face again. That's purely anecdotal. It was quite some
time later when I read that numbness of the face is a typical reaction
to the chemicals in fabric softeners.

Oddly enough, I finally learned about MCS accidentally through
my coworkers. One of them came to me and said, "You ought to see
what's going up on the bulletin board." When I went to look I found
a column clipped from a newspaper, taking to task a woman named
Julia Kendall, who was filing a lawsuit against a department store
for mailing printed materials scented with fragrances to her home.
The columnist commented that the fragrance issue was going too
far. One of my coworkers had highlighted that remark and added a
note, "Barb, this means you!" Someone else had posted a note that
said, "Barb has company." I didn't even read the whole column. I
left it there and posted a note that said, "Coughing is asthma and it
hurts." Shortly thereafter I returned to find the column and all the
notes had been tossed in the trash. I pulled the newspaper clipping
out of the garbage, shook off the coffee grounds, took it back to my
office and dried it out. After it dried I read the entire article and started
to shake. Something in me resonated with Julia Kendall.

Sitting in my office clutching the newspaper article, I picked up
the phone and called Julia. She said, "What you have is MCS." That
was the beginning of my learning process, and a great relief to finally
confirm I wasn't the only one with this problem.

Julia mentored me, provided me with resources and mailed me
a lot of information. At that time she was working on a handout

describing the effects of the thirty-one most common chemicals found in fragrances. She put that together from an EPA report released in '91, and from information she got from the MSDS (Material Safety and Data Sheets) for every one of those chemicals. She became well known for that piece of work before she died of cancer.

One of the things Julia sent me was a brochure she'd made called "Making Sense of Scents," explaining the effects of fragrances on people with MCS. I posted it on the bulletin board at work in an attempt to inform the staff that this was what I had, that I wasn't so weird after all, and that it could happen to them. I didn't want anybody else to have to go through what I had been through. Someone came along and wrote on it, "Get a life!" I wrote back, "I have a life and I plan to continue having a life." That stayed up for a month or better, much to my surprise.

With the "Get a Life" incident I began a practice that helped me to cope with harassment. I decided that any time one of these "hateful hurts" was thrown at me I would treat it like manure, which happens to make things grow nicely. I wrote a letter to Julia and told her that every time I was a recipient of harassment I would send her money to help her pay for copying and mailing MCS information out to other people. So I used my painful experiences as a way to spread the word.

The same year that I learned about MCS, our agency was required to begin training in the Americans with Disabilities Act. I learned enough from the training to know I had a right to reasonable accommodations in the workplace. I requested that low–VOC paints be used whenever the walls were painted. I asked that notices for meetings contain a request for those in attendance to refrain from wearing scents. And I asked that the use of fragrances in the office environment be kept to a minimum. They wouldn't do any of that or anything else that I asked. So, I accommodated myself by purchasing my own masks, respirator and oxygen tank, and an air filter for my office. After that the harassment escalated. For a while someone was spraying something that smelled like manure outside my office door every morning. I kept my door closed, so it didn't bother me at all but it bothered everyone else.

One of the things that happens to a lot of people with MCS in the workplace is that we are cut off from the rest of the staff and ostracized under the guise of accommodations. That's what happened in my case. My human resources manager convinced my doctor that my best interests were the priority in a decision made to move me to an office by myself. What she didn't mention was that the office had no windows that opened; it was two floors away from my staff, next to the cafeteria and a conference room where crowds of scented people gathered; it was near a door where smokers stood to smoke their cigarettes, and near a public restroom. It also turned out that diesel fumes came in through the door and through the ventilation system and got trapped in my office, fiberglass shards were falling from the ceiling, and solvent fumes were coming through the air vents—a fact which they denied for a long time. I knew they were setting up problems for me, hoping I would get a belly full and leave.

I had asked to telecommunicate from home, because that would have been a reasonable accommodation under the ADA. But they said no. Instead, I telecommunicated from two floors away. In essence, I was stripped of all my job responsibilities.

I moved my things out of my old office in a shopping cart. When I went back to get what was still remaining, some of my coworkers were chortling and cahorting in there. When I walked in they went out the other door. I felt so betrayed. It felt like a knife going in with a twist. I thought: Damn it to hell! That's what my mother always said when things got this bad.

In that kind of situation, you either stick it out or quit. I decided to stick it out, because I actually liked my job and most of the people I worked with really liked me. One woman in particular offered her support. Others told me they, too, were experiencing sick building symptoms while at work. But everybody was watching their own career ladders and had to be careful. I didn't want to put anyone else in jeopardy. During the last two years I was forbidden to use the word "fragrance," and my lunch buddy was told never to mention the word either.

What happened to me in my workplace is happening to people all over the country. My vow was that I would do the best job I possibly could while I was there, but after I retired I would do everything in my power to make it better for anyone else going through what I went through. For starters, I joined the toxics committee of the Sierra Club, and worked with another member to get a resolution passed to discourage the use of fragranced products in all public places. We were fully prepared for some resistance, but when we made the presentation they actually made the language stronger and it was passed. It begins, "The Sierra Club discourages the use of fragranced products and encourages the use of fragrance-free products in all public places. They advocate educating people, employers, employees, businesses and the media about the insidious nature of toxic chemicals in fragranced products and their role in associated disabilities for both users and secondhand recipients alike."

That gives me chills, my dear!

Pacific Northwest Stories

Were it not for the fact that the great heroes and spiritual leaders of mankind have spoken in mystic terms it would be easy to discount their experience as insane.—From *Ordinary People as Monks and Mystics* by Marsha Sinetar

Herbert Whitish
Shoalwater Bay Indian
Reservation, Washington

Looking at Herbert Whitish, chairman and health director of the Shoalwater Bay Tribe, you'd never dream he's ill. Members of his tribe and family have no idea he suffers with chronic fatigue, chemical sensitivities, and loss of his ability to participate in activities he once enjoyed. The day his photo was taken for this publication, he was too ill to participate in the interview, which was later accomplished by telephone.

Two passions shape his life: his family and his tribe. His sense of duty provides him with the will to persevere despite poor health.

Raised mostly in Seattle, Herb moved with his parents to the reservation a few years before he left for college at Western Washington University. After college he worked as a biologist for the State of Washington and the Northwest Indian Fisheries Commission, then returned to the reservation when his mother died to help his father operate his grocery store. Herb, with his wife, has continued the family business, along with his tribal responsibilities. They have four children between the ages of nineteen and twenty-two, and grandchildren.

I look at my people and they have so many needs. I have to keep going in order to help them achieve what they rightfully should have. My work and my family have kept me going through this illness, through the days when I find myself so tired I fall asleep in the office.

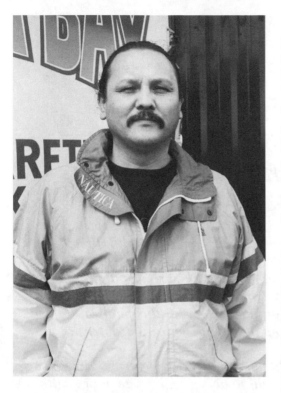

Out of ninety tribal people who live here, five have chronic fatigue. That's a pretty large group for a small area. You wonder why mostly reservation people are sick in this area, although we don't know for sure that there aren't a lot of other people in the area who are also ill. All we can talk about is what we know, and what we know is tribal.

About 1990 we experienced a cluster of losses on the reservation, including several pregnancies in various stages, and a one-year-old child. So we started collecting anecdotal evidence to try to determine what was going on. We discovered a majority of our women having adverse reproductive outcomes. Indian Health Services said we didn't have a problem. So, we spent three years lobbying Congress to get money for a study to determine the causes of our problems. It was believed that one possibility could be chemical contamination, because chemicals are used on properties all around the reservation. The cranberry industry uses chemicals, the oyster industry uses chemicals, the lumber industry uses chemicals on their trees, and the State of Washington uses chemicals to control a non-native grass taking over the bay, and along the roads.

The Environmental Protection Agency did a study of the cranberry drainage area and the tidelands area where people swim and gather clams. They determined that the chemicals in the cranberry ditches exceeded federal and state guidelines, but they could not make a cause and effect link from the chemicals to what was happening on the reservation. It's such a political issue. If you say anything, somebody accuses you of trying to negatively affect their livelihood. You can't blame them. To prove there is a connection at all between the chemical usage and the health problems on the reservation is difficult.

I first became aware that I was ill six or eight years ago. I went from enjoying an active lifestyle to being constantly tired. My bones ached and my muscles hurt and I had headaches all the time. I got to the point where I'd fall asleep at all times of the day—and still do. It's kind of a scary feeling, because I can't control it. It was difficult to realize I couldn't even work at times. I'm so tired right now that I can hardly reflect my thoughts. I think it's going to be one of those days when I'm going to have to take a nap.

When I'm out in public I have to avoid perfumes. Certain scents are overwhelming to me. My sinuses instantly begin to hurt, I get a severe headache and a nauseous feeling rushes over me. It's unbearable at times.

I kept going to all the doctors around here because I consistently felt terrible, and they couldn't explain anything. They kept alluding to the idea that maybe I was suffering from something mental. It wasn't until I went to a doctor up in Seattle that they found I had the Epstein-Barr virus.

That was the most depressing part, when I couldn't find an answer. You begin to question yourself. You don't want to go to a doctor again for fear they're just going to tell you you're losing your grip. If you're told something enough times you start to believe it. I started to wonder, was this a result of depression from losing my parents so close to each other? Was it a guilt process of some kind because my behavior was less than exemplary in my earlier life? To find out it wasn't anything of that nature was a big relief.

During that period of not understanding what was going on, the will to get back to the way I was before kept me going. It was a big relief to finally have an answer, although so little was known about the cause of this illness. There were so many theories about what it was, so I really didn't get any straight answers as to what causes it or what you can do about it. Everything was new and fairly experimental. Nobody had any definitive answers, and I don't know if they do today. Finally I resigned myself to the fact that my quality of life was not going to be as it was in the past, and I was just going to have to do the best I could. I realized this probably is never going to change. I quit dwelling on it because I realized there's not a great deal I can do about it. Now I put my mind on my work and try not to think about the illness.

You have to come to the realization that you can't do everything you did previously. But you can't let this illness push you to the point where you've got to quit. The worst thing that can happen is to let it completely defeat you. Because once you do quit, where are you going to go from there?

There are always resources available. It might be a confidante, somebody to talk to, like my wife was after I was diagnosed. That helped me to start dealing with the fact that I had chronic fatigue. To me, everybody's got an internal resource, too. The mind is a wonderful thing and can do many things for you. You have to start training your mind to get over the obstacles.

My parents taught me that you can't expect people to do things for you. Whatever life gives you, you have to deal with it. It's not somebody else's problem. I believed this was my problem and I had to find ways to deal with it. I'm not rich, so I had to keep working. I had to work through the issue that if I was going to continue to work I'd have to figure out ways to deal with being chronically ill.

The last thing I wanted was for people to treat me differently or to show sympathy. If people were trying to make allowances for me, I wouldn't feel like I was earning my keep. That would have been more harmful to my peace of mind than anything. So I decided it was best to not say anything about it to anybody, to just go on with what I've got to do. I've never told anyone except my wife. She has helped me through a lot by being there all the time. When I was really down or so tired I couldn't do anything, she'd fill in for me. She'd pull the weight. Bringing up three sons and a daughter, a lot of the burden fell on her. She helps me at the store and lets me nap a lot, and we get through.

Now that I've learned how to deal with my illness in a way that people wouldn't even realize anything was going on, I don't care if others know. I'm not going to make a point of telling people because they might start treating me differently. I hope, now that people are more familiar with chronic fatigue, they wouldn't leap to assumptions or worry that it might be contagious. It's not contagious. It's probably nothing that's ever going to kill me. And it's not something that's just in my head.

The hardest part for me is the inability to do as much as I used to. I used to be very active. I loved to drive automobiles, and could drive for hours and hours and not get tired. I'd drive all over the state. Now it's a major chore just to get into Seattle and back. And I don't have the energy to walk on the beach or that kind of thing. I work, go home and go to sleep. Even that is difficult at times.

This illness doesn't have to destroy your entire life. There are ways to cope, whether that is of a spiritual nature or a work ethic.

Believing in the Smokehouse helps me to cope. I don't know if you'd call it a religion, it's a way of life. People come from all different tribes. These are people who care about other people. Their whole philosophy is to follow a good lifestyle. Being with other people, especially at the Smokehouse, lifts my spirits.

I'm not a touchy-feely kind of person. Most of the time I can't tell people what my feelings are, but I can help by doing the things I'm doing as chairman and health director. I have a lot of faults. But one thing I do know how to do is work hard. So every time I feel like quitting—and there have been many times since I've been sick—I ask myself: What would I do? Would I just lay around and feel sorry for myself? That was no kind of an answer either. I put everything I've got into this job and my family. I believe that defines who I am as a person. I try to lead by example. That's why I couldn't succumb to this illness. I just had to find another way to do it. It's taken some adjustments to compensate for the inability to do things I used to do.

People depend on me, and I think I'm doing something that is worthy. I have an overwhelming need to help. That makes it more difficult for me to allow this to beat me. There are times when it would be so much easier to just quit and roll over. I'm not going to let that happen. My parents taught me to keep plugging away until the day I die, otherwise I don't live up to my potential. When I was very young my father went to Alaska so he could earn enough money to move us out of the housing projects in the south end of Seattle. He didn't like having his family living in that area, so he sacrificed a great deal to make life better for his family. My mom did the same thing. She worked sixteen and eighteen hours a day shaking crab and that kind of thing so she could make my life better. Those lessons weren't talked about, but I could see how hard they worked and believed in that kind of life. My parents worked until the day they died. When I needed that kind of an ethic, it was there. It's funny how those things you never paid much attention to at the time come back and give you a reminder that there are ways to deal with difficulties. There is hope.

Alanna and Mariah Ahern Bainbridge Island, Washington

Three words come to mind when I recall my meeting with then-fifteen-year-old Alanna Ahern: articulate, mature and delightful. This young woman clearly views difficult life events as challenges rather than problems. Suffering from asthma and allergies since birth could easily have resulted in poor self-esteem and a self-image associated with illness. Instead she has developed a picture of herself as a person who is powerful and effective, and one who overcomes adversity.

Born in Arizona, Alanna's asthma was so severe that she was sick almost constantly and rarely left the house as a small child. Her family moved to the Pacific Northwest when she was five, hoping she could breathe better in a different environment. Alanna was in the fourth grade when her face swelled so severely in school one day that her mother, Ka'ren, began an investigation into the cause, an investigation of many months' duration. Meanwhile, Alanna's respiratory problems worsened and she complained of feeling spacey and detached from her body while in school. Her doctor informed them that she was experiencing symptoms of chemical exposure. Ka'ren discovered that the children were exposed to solvents and other chemicals used to remodel the school while classes were in session. Eventually, other parents joined the effort, numerous government agencies and the media were involved, and a lawsuit was settled out of court for damages suffered by another student who was chemically injured.

Through many hours of consultations with experts in toxicology, medicine and environmental health, Ka'ren learned about MCS, and finally realized that even she and her other daughter Mariah, age nine at interview, were reacting to chemicals from fragrances and other sources. It explained to her why Alanna's colds and sore throats so often developed into pneumonia or bronchitis, and why she experienced asthma attacks for no apparent reason. This awakening also prompted her to examine her own history of chemical exposures.

Other than an allergy to dairy as an infant, Ka'ren experienced no unusual health problems until adolescence. Then quite often she could hardly stay awake in school. In retrospect she questions the connection between her fatigue and her family's move to a farm where pesticides were in heavy use. Her fond childhood memories now seem tragic as she recalls watching airplanes zoom across the fields dropping pesticides. She ran through the clouds of chemicals with her dog, and also rode with her brother when he sprayed pesticides from a tank attached to the back of a car. She remembers the peppery smell of the chemicals they sprayed, a smell she found pleasant and intoxicating. Although she was an outstanding student, she missed a lot of school due to chronic fatigue, colds and infections, which she now attributes to chemical injury. From her research she concluded that many chemicals stored in her body tissue were passed to Alanna during breastfeeding. She believes this, and a genetic predisposition for allergies, explains Alanna's susceptibility to MCS.

Mariah also inherited a susceptibility to allergies and asthma, but did not acquire the same dose of toxins from breastfeeding. (Studies indicate that the greatest burden of toxins in the mother's body are off-loaded during the first six months of breastfeeding.) She was a strong child with no history of chronic illness until an incident occurred in her school. Because the electricity had gone out, the toilets weren't flushing. When the toilets were full of urine the janitor poured chlorine into them in an attempt to reduce the odor. The mixture of urine and chlorine proved to be a toxic combination. Ka'ren arrived at the school for volunteer work just as the children were dismissed from class. She detected the toxic odor and tried to protect the children by keeping them out of the restrooms. As she stood in the hallway directing the children to go outdoors to safety, Mariah ran past her, directly into the restroom. Mariah's nose, throat and lungs were burned from inhaling the fumes, and she developed asthma.

Since learning about the effects of chemicals found in ordinary products used at home and in school, Ka'ren has led a crusade and joined forces with the Washington Toxics Coalition to make the schools in her community safer for children. Largely due to their efforts the Bainbridge Island School District recently adopted an Integrated Pest Management program to minimize the use of pesticides on school property. The groundskeepers were delighted, according to Ka'ren. The next step she hopes the school will take is to adopt

*a complete nontoxic product policy and a centralized purchasing
program so that the same nontoxic products are used in every school.
Once created and adopted, this program could provide a model for
schools nationwide, a model that will reduce costs and protect children from unnecessary chemical exposures.*

Alanna

I don't think of myself as chemically sensitive now. That's a
chapter of my life that I think I've pretty much dealt with. Even a
year or two ago I couldn't have run down the street without getting
asthma. Now I run stairs and jog miles and miles. My life has changed
a lot.

Our family is so informed that I don't have to worry about chemicals in our house. And we eat right and take a lot of vitamins, so
even if sometimes I do run into perfume or something, it won't bother
me now as much as it would have maybe two years ago. I don't think
about it too much, but I'm cautious. I'm alert every day, and that
pretty much keeps me well. But occasionally I get a wake-up call.
Sometimes I get rashes or hives, or I'll get an instant sore throat when
I'm exposed to certain hair products and that kind of thing. I get
a migraine about once a month, which jolts me back to the reality
that I have to deal with this. Or, if I don't want to ask my friends
to not wear perfume, and I just ignore it, I get sick. But I don't dwell
on it.

I've had asthma and allergies all of my life, but I wasn't aware
of my chemical sensitivity until I was in the fourth grade. It was right
after spring break. They had started some remodeling in my school
during the break, and it was still in progress when we went back.
There was wet adhesive all over the floors, and brand new paint and
carpeting in the classrooms. I was sitting in class when my teacher
looked at me and said, "Did you have dental work? Your face is so
puffy!" I thought: What is she talking about? When I came home and
walked in the house my mother screamed, "What's wrong with you?"
I said, "What do you mean?" She said, "Your face is so swollen!"
I didn't understand why.

That's the day my mom started investigating. We didn't know
anything about MCS at that point and had to educate ourselves.

I continued going to school before we realized what was happening. I got really sick, although that wasn't unusual for me. Even before all this I was never a student with perfect attendance; I missed school a lot because of allergies, asthma and a weak immune system. But we couldn't figure out why I was coming down with more colds and infections than usual. It would start out like a regular cold, with a sore throat and stuffy nose. But then it would progress into pneumonia and bronchitis. I've had pneumonia too many times to count.

By then other people were complaining, too. It wasn't just me. Other kids were getting headaches, stomachaches and more colds and infections. When my mom and some of the other parents figured out that chemical exposures were making us ill, they were pretty angry. But there wasn't any one person to be angry at. The school administrators should have been more informed, but they didn't know. It wasn't really their fault, and they were nice people. You couldn't be angry with the construction workers. They were just doing their jobs and didn't know what effects chemicals were having on the kids.

By the time I was in the fifth grade my mom was educated and my doctor helped her to realize I couldn't go to school in that building. She pulled me out of school and got a tutor to work with me at home. That was a pretty hard time for me. I didn't want to be pulled out of school; nobody does at that age. School is your only connection to a social life. So, I wasn't happy about it but I knew it was the right decision. The school wasn't a safe place for me, or for anyone, for that matter. When I stopped going to that school I started the process of getting healthy.

I lost contact with many friends. My best friends came to visit, but they couldn't really understand because it wasn't happening to them. I would sometimes visit my class, like on Valentine's Day. But it was hard for me to accept when I couldn't participate in the class play and other fun things they did. I got pretty upset at those times, and cried a lot. Yet I understood.

Once I went to a birthday party at an outdoor pool. The chlorine was so overpowering to me that I got really sick and weak. I told my mom, "Don't *ever* let me go back to that pool again!"

Sometimes I felt pretty hopeless, like when I was supposed to go back to school at the end of fifth grade. I got sick and couldn't go back that day. That happened twice. I thought, God, is this my life? Am I always going to be this sick? I thought I would always have to be homeschooled.

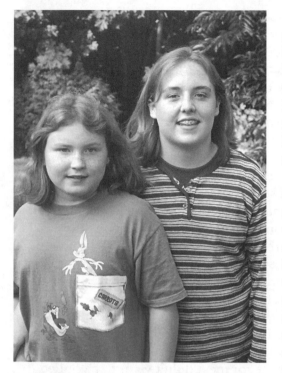

Mariah (left) and Alanna Ahern

Having asthma, allergies and chemical sensitivities can be a very deadly combination. During the peak of my sensitivity I really didn't leave the house much. I didn't go to movies or shopping. Things like that just weren't a part of my life.

It's not fun to be different than everyone else. There is stigma with that. Other kids wondered why I was out of school so much. They didn't see me when I was sick, so it was hard to understand. Some of them even thought I wasn't really sick. That's the kind of remarks I heard even from some of my friends. Some kids talked behind my back. I didn't blame them because they've never had to deal with it. All of my friends were really healthy.

My family helped me to get through it; I wasn't dealing with it by myself. It took a while for my dad to understand, because he's a big healthy-like-a-horse kind of guy. He's a natural kind of guy, though, too. Even before we knew about chemical sensitivity our family never used products with a lot of fragrance or perfume. It's been Dr. Bronner's all the way. We're brown rice and broccoli people. My family is very supportive and has helped me all the way. It's a family commitment.

In the sixth grade we had a brand new middle school. That was trying, too. My mom worked with them a lot to make sure they were using safer products. But I still had problems. I remember the day we first toured the new school. The odor from the floor in the new gymnasium was so pungent and strong that kids were coughing. We knew I could never use the gym. I went to study hall, things like that, during that period. There were vinyl wallboards everywhere, and for a while we used portable, manufactured classrooms that were very caustic. I got by, but I was not healthy. I felt spacey and detached from my body from the fumes. One time I walked into a classroom where a teacher had used a graffiti remover an hour earlier. I knew immediately I had to get out of the room, my brain was affected that quick. I went out to my locker and could not remember the combination, and I felt terrified. I've experienced some memory loss from that period. There's a lot that I don't remember, like math. I should have learned pre-algebra in the sixth grade, but I had to take it all over again as a freshman because I didn't remember any of it.

In high school I have to be healthy to keep up my grades. In my freshman year I decided I was going to be on the swim team. I love to swim, so I decided that was what I was going to do. My best friend lives across the street and she's on the swim team, too. We do it together.

The community raised the funds for an ozonator for the pool. It aerates the pool and they don't have to use so much chlorine. I'm really happy about that, because I'm not getting as much chlorine into my system. The whole community wanted it. They're more educated because of people like my mom. After they get educated they realize what has to be done.

I'm pretty consumed by school, especially right now, when I'm on the swim team. I swim six days a week. It's very involved. I love it, but sometimes I don't want to go to practice. It's really good for me, though. I'm a lot stronger because of it. My lungs are much healthier. I've built up my immune system. That's partly why chemicals don't bother me so much now.

I have to be really careful though. An exposure to chemicals can be too much, especially when I'm active in a sport. I'm just cautious—that's my motto. But I do what all fifteen-year-olds like to do, I hang out with my friends. I even go shopping with my friends a lot, but I avoid the perfume aisles and other things that make me sick.

All my teachers and my coach understand that I'm chemically sensitive. The nurse at our school has educated them. So they look out for me, and let me know if they're going to use something that might bother me. That helps, because I don't like to advertise that I'm chemically sensitive. I don't like to draw too much attention to myself. But I will speak up and take care of myself when I need to. I won't sit there and let stuff happen to me. If someone is going to use a product that is not safe for me, I'll evacuate the area. I've had to learn how to speak up for myself. My mom pushed me into it because, when she sent me off to school, she had to trust me with my life. She told me I *had* to let my teachers know if anything bothered me. I was pretty young to be responsible for it myself. Now it's second nature, and one of my greatest strengths. I think it's pretty important for anyone, because if you don't speak up for yourself you're not going to get what you need.

I take care of myself by moving, or leaving the room, if someone is spraying something. If I need to, I say, "This is making me sick and I need to leave the room." But I don't always have to announce it to the world. I take care of myself more freely now than I used to.

Most of the time I don't have to deal with MCS. My allergies are more of a problem at this point. I'm allergic to dairy and other foods, and cats. I'm allergic to many things. I have to think of that kind of stuff before I go to someone's house or spend the night with a friend.

Strength of mind has enabled me to overcome a lot and get to where I am now. I don't think of MCS as something that will hold me back. I want others with MCS to know that it doesn't have to control your life. If you take care of yourself you get stronger, and then you don't have to deal with it as much. I'm much stronger than I used to be. That's pretty encouraging.

MCS is not as horrible as you may think. I'm glad I understand this important issue, and it's nice to be able to talk about it to groups. I've met a lot of interesting people and learned something about politics. I was on the *Northwest Afternoon* show with Dr. Doris Rapp, and I've been able to help my mom with activist work. For years my mother was consumed with working for the environment. Now, as others take over that work, she doesn't always have to be on the battlefield.

A lot of companies are coming out with fragrance-free products, and you see a lot of brochures, now, for meetings that are "fragrance-free." People are beginning to understand the effects of fragrances and other chemicals, and that is a direct result of people like my mother. They're really pioneers. More people are saying they get sick from fragrances, and it's starting to make a difference.

Mariah

My friends sometimes go and run and I can't run with them because I have asthma and it's hard for me to breathe. I ask my friends if they could wait for me, and usually they are pretty good about that. Lots of people like me and they don't want to lose my friendship. My friends Delsa and Electra always make sure they're not leaving me behind.

When I meet someone I have to tell them to please not wear any perfume or hair gel or anything like that around me. I have to tell them a whole bunch of stuff and they have to understand before we can be friends, because its really hard if someone doesn't understand and they wear hair spray or something, or they don't wait up for me. When I smell perfume it's hard for me to breathe and it feels like my throat is closing. It's hard, because a lot of people wear it. My mom talked to my teachers to make sure they don't wear perfume. It's mainly a problem at the beginning of the year when the teachers forget that kids are allergic to it. Lots of kids in my school have asthma.

Sometimes I feel like my friends are different, and I wish that I could do what they're doing. But I can't. Since I'm allergic I can't pet cats or guinea pigs and some other animals. If I touch them, I break out in hives or I can't breathe. I can't go to a friend's house if they have cats. That's really hard. My friend Electra has cats and I can't go over to her house. We always play at my house.

There are a lot of foods I can't eat because I'm allergic. I can't eat dairy so I can't drink milk or eat macaroni and cheese. I'm careful about what I eat. I can't eat kiwi. Once I just touched a kiwi and I broke out in hives.

I would like people to understand that I am normal, I just can't do some of the things that they can do.

Peggy Kadey
Whidbey Island, Washington

In August 1995 Peggy Kadey, then fifty-two, accidentally left a pot of beans on the stove and went shopping with her husband, Ron. When they returned the house was full of smoke. A restoration

company came to repair the damage with ozone. Peggy and her hus-
band assumed the process was safe. When they were told they could
return home, an ozone machine was still running in their bedroom.
Although the door was sealed, the ozone circulated through the heat-
ing ducts in the house. While talking on the telephone immediately
upon returning home, Peggy was poisoned by the ozone as it poured
out of the register located directly under her stool. A series of attempts
to make the house safe again only injured her further.

For a long time Peggy believed that her injury was temporary.
In reality she had developed a chronic, progressive illness, so severe
that her doctors feared for her life on several occasions. After dozens
of medical tests she learned that the mucous membrane throughout
her respiratory system was badly damaged, her immune system was
so severely impaired that she was at great risk of developing cancer,
her brain and liver were affected, her blood was loaded with toxic
chemicals, and she could no longer tolerate even extremely low lev-
els of chemical exposures. A short time later she developed breast
cancer.

Chemotherapy used to treat cancer is toxic by almost anyone's
standards. How would it affect someone like Peggy, who experiences
life-threatening reactions to even low-level chemical exposures? There
are no answers. Peggy believes chemotherapy or surgery could be
fatal for her, because her lungs burn and airways can close even from
exposure to fragrances and other ordinary products. She has chosen
to treat her cancer with a non-chemical, non-invasive alternative pro-
gram, and her trust in God.

When this interview took place she and Ron had recently moved
to a rural location to minimize her exposures to toxins in the city.
She spends most of her time alone or with Ron, because exposure
to other people can cause her to be incapacitated for days. One of
the places she longs to go is to a theater to see the movie Life Is
Beautiful.

Peggy has two children and five grandchildren.

———————

There are times when I'm here all alone, day after day, week
after week, when I don't see anybody except my husband. I think:
How can I be useful? I have a very strong faith. I pray. And I talk
to God. I tell him, okay, I gave my life to you once, now what are

you going to do with it? I want to give something to this world. I want to give back for having had a life, for being allowed to be on this planet. I feel a need to do something for mankind.

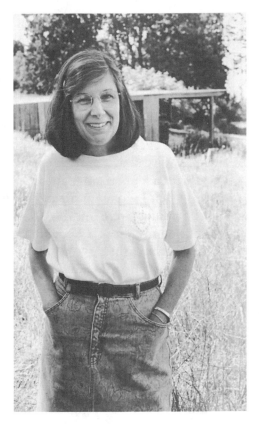

I can't believe this is happening to me all because I left a pot of beans on the stove. Unfortunately, it is very real.

I completely trusted the guy from the restoration company when he told us that the ozone would destroy the smoke particles and make the house fresh-smelling just like the outdoors. He told me that ozone is so volatile that it changes right back into oxygen. When we were told it was okay to reoccupy the house, we came home and found a note on the door. It said there was still an ozone generator running in the bedroom but it was okay because the door was sealed, and that if we needed to go in there all we had to do was unplug the machine and wait a few minutes before entering the room. I figured they knew what they were doing and there was no reason for me to be fearful.

The smoke smell was gone, and there was a real sweet smell in the house. I got right on the phone and started calling people to let them know we were back home. I kept calling people and pretty soon I started feeling ill. My nose and mouth felt really dry and I could feel a sensation in my airways, like something was moving along my airways heading for my lungs. I know this sounds weird. It *was* weird, and creepy. I called the restoration company and they said, "Pull the plug on the generator, open all the windows and get out of the house real quick. Stay away until this evening, and then it will be okay." That's when it hit me that they'd tried to secure the bedroom by sealing the door, but probably hadn't closed off the ducts in the room. When I asked them what they'd done about the ducts in the bedroom they said, "Nothing." That ozone had been pumping right into my face while I talked on the phone. But they assured me I would be fine, that a little dryness was nothing to worry about.

That night my lungs were still burning and I felt sick, but I thought it was temporary. Ron's aunt and uncle had planned to spend the night with us, and half an hour after they arrived they started complaining of dry throats. So we drank some juice and went to bed, thinking everything would be fine in the morning. Aunt Margie and Uncle Wilson are brother and sister, so Margie slept with me on a bed with a latex foam mattress. Ron and Wilson slept in other rooms.

When I woke up my mouth was burning, my nose was burning and my lungs were burning. I could hardly breathe. When I bent over to put on my slippers I couldn't get any air. I stood up and could take only tiny breaths. I woke up my husband and tried to tell him what was going on. I told him I had to get out of there. Wilson and Margie left right away because they sensed there was something terribly wrong in the house.

What we learned much later is that ozone gets trapped in fabrics and is released when the fabrics are disturbed, and it changes foam and other substances into toxic compounds. So, the bed I slept in poisoned me further and there was ozone trapped in all of our upholstered furniture and on other fabrics. Aunt Margie doesn't claim to have any long-term effects from sleeping on that bed, but she no longer wears perfume or uses the same cleaning products she used to use because now they make her cough. Thank goodness she didn't also have the initial massive ozone exposure that I did.

Our grandchildren were coming to spend that day with us, so we took them to the zoo so we could spend the day outside, still thinking I'd be fine. But all I could do at the park was sit on a bench. I couldn't even carry my purse. My doctor didn't know what was happening to me, and told me to call the occupational medicine department at a local hospital. I called and was put on a three-week waiting list for an appointment, and a nurse told me to start keeping a record of every symptom, every call I made, everything that was going on. She told me not to stop looking for help.

That night we went to a hotel, and the next day I started making calls from my bed. The first person I contacted, at the health department, said, "Your symptoms are consistent with a high level exposure to ozone." I called the EPA and anybody else I was referred to in every conversation.

When I finally went to see a specialist in occupational medicine, I told him my mouth and lungs and all my airways were burning, and that even the air conditioning in our car made my lungs burn. I was told the ozone had done this to me but that it was temporary and I would be fine. So I put up with continuous pain for weeks, thinking it was only a matter of time until I healed. I couldn't even drink orange juice because the acid burned my tongue and the roof of my mouth. I started getting nosebleeds because the ozone had dissolved the mucous membrane in my nose.

That doctor told me that all the carpeting in our house, all the fabrics, all our clothes, and all the furniture would have to be cleaned to get rid of the hydrocarbons left behind by the smoke. He also told me that ozone changes the environment and can cause formaldehyde levels to be higher.

All of our clothes were sent to a cleaners and we hired a different restoration company to come and clean everything in the house while we stayed in a hotel. I told the supervisor of this company that only nontoxic, natural products could be used in my house. She assured me that would be no problem, and that in three days I would be able to move back home. But when I walked in to inspect the house I could actually taste the chemicals they'd used and my mouth and lungs burned. Someone from our insurance company found a spray bottle they'd left behind in our rec room closet. That's how we found out they had used strong solvents. Eventually they came back and tried everything to make the house safe. They scrubbed with TSP and they scrubbed with vinegar. They tried everything in the world, but nothing worked. This house that had been custom built for us was now a toxic waste dump.

In November the insurance company said they wouldn't pay for anything more, that the house was perfectly fine, but we were never able to occupy the house again. We rented a room in a friends' house and had to put our house on the market. It took a year for us to restore that house, out of our own pockets, before we could sell it.

My health continued to deteriorate. When I tried to go shopping I got so nauseated I had to leave the store. I couldn't add numbers. I didn't know where to go or what to do. I still didn't know what was happening to me. Someone finally referred me to a doctor who told me I had a chemical injury and there were probably solvents in my bloodstream. I said, "No, I don't think so. They told me at the hospital that I would be fine."

I had some tests done and there *were* solvents in my blood, the same ones that showed up on air quality tests done in my house. The doctor had never seen a benzene level as high as I had in my blood. These solvents can cause cancer and brain damage, so I got into an intensive detoxification program in a medical clinic.

We had bought another house with the help of relatives. I felt like everything in the world was making me sick. My brain was so dysfunctional and chemicals were affecting me so badly that I couldn't drive a car, I couldn't read, I couldn't remember my phone number or address, and I lost my sense of direction. That's when my doctors started to teach us what it means to make a house "safe." We had to get rid of all our clothes—four closets full—that had just been dry cleaned. We had to get rid of all the cleaning products, colognes, nail polish. All that stuff.

My brain was so overloaded with chemicals at that time that I experienced three suicidal episodes. The air outside was too toxic for me, the air inside was too toxic, and the inside of my car was toxic. I couldn't think. I didn't know what to do. I could see no reason to live. There was no place to go.

On one of those occasions I picked up the phone and called my dad and said, "Whatever you do, don't hang up! If you hang up I'm not going to make it. I'm out of control." I kept him on the phone for an hour, screaming and crying. I had no control over it.

Another time I called my sister when that happened. And the last time my husband was here to experience it.

I don't think my doctors even knew what to do at that point. They kept telling me to just stay in my bedroom with an air filter going. They told me I just had to wait it out. My husband, my children and other family members all said, "You've got a lot to live for. We all love you. You have grandchildren. You've got to get better." Their love gave me just enough hope to help me get through that crisis period.

A turning point came when I finally detected that I was reacting to ordinary things in our house. Every time I walked near the window blinds I felt like they were knocking me over and I could taste chemicals in my mouth. I didn't know if my husband would believe me or not, but in my desperation I ripped down all the blinds in the house. When he came home all the blinds were outside in the garbage. After that I noticed a chemical taste in my mouth every time I opened a kitchen cupboard. We figured out that it was from the formaldehyde in the particleboard, so Ron replaced all the particleboard in the house with wire shelving. All the fiberglass screens were replaced with aluminum. We stopped using the gas fireplace. And we had a HEPA filter built into the heating system. I also put carbon filters over all the heat ducts, and started running air filters twenty-four hours a day.

I also figured out that certain foods were contributing to my brain fog, so I avoided those and started making my breakfast from an immune support recipe I was given, with milk thistle, lecithin, flax seed and all kinds of things in it. Gradually, my total load of chemicals was reduced and I got my brain back. Then there was *so* much hope!

That's when I started my research to try to understand what was happening to me. I called the library and started having books delivered to my home. I still didn't believe this would be long-term. I couldn't understand why I was in so much pain or why my mouth and lungs were still burning even when I wasn't having trouble breathing, or why I became deathly ill for no apparent reason. If I went out to an appointment, the next day or two I'd experience diarrhea, vomiting and chills. Sometimes I was completely non-functional for days.

Once I got so severely sick going into one hospital for testing that I didn't get past the front entrance. I had to leave and have the test done at another place. And when my son was in a hospital for surgery, I desperately wanted to see him so I went to the hospital for just a few minutes, and it took me days to recover. I've been through so much. Several times I wasn't sure I was going to live. At one point I lost so much weight that I was down to what I weighed in junior high school. And one time my airways completely closed from an exposure to perfume. My doctors pulled me through. There were many days when I was too sick to go to their office, but they were always there for me by telephone. And I received a lot of telephone support from the nurse in my doctor's office.

It was in September of last year that I discovered a lump in my breast. I felt it when I was lying in bed next to my husband with one arm up over my head. I cried all that weekend. I thought about my options, and about my doctor telling me my liver was so damaged. Every time Ron spoke or asked me a question, I cried.

I saw a doctor who aspirated cells from my breast and confirmed they were malignant. The procedure was done without any

medication because I didn't think I could even tolerate a local anesthetic. The doctor recommended a lumpectomy plus radiation, or
a radical mastectomy. I told her I didn't think any of those were
options for me because I'm so chemically injured. I got sick just walking through her waiting room where there were people wearing
perfume.

I told the doctor I was going to Hawaii for my thirty-fifth wedding anniversary, and that I would do a lot of thinking and give her
my decision when I came back.

Ron had free tickets to fly to Hawaii, and we had found chemical-free homes to stay in on Maui and Kauai. Ron and I had been
working with my environmental doctor and a respiratory therapist
to find a way for me to make the trip safely. A friend of mine—a
nurse—went with us to the airport to help me get to the plane. The
level of perfume in the airport was so high that, even on oxygen, I
felt terribly sick and begged Ron to take me back to the car. But I
was in a wheelchair and they insisted that I was going to Hawaii.
On the plane I used the oxygen with my own stainless steel tubing
and ceramic mask.

So much planning and preparation went into making that trip
possible for me. We even found a rental car company that agreed
to steam clean a car and wash the whole inside over and over with
vinegar until it worked for me. We were in Hawaii for three weeks.
We didn't go to public places but every day we went to a different
beach.

I did a lot of thinking about my cancer treatment options while
I was there. The surgeon called me as soon as I was back from our
trip. I told her my decision was to try natural, alternative treatments,
and to keep an eye on the tumor. I told her I would be really concerned if it grew to the size of an egg. She said, "When it gets to the
size of an egg it will be terminal and there will be nothing I can do
for you." I said, "Okay, but I'm going to try alternative programs."

Ron was really upset about my decision. He and other family
members have tried to talk me into having surgery. They were going
to drag me in to have something done. But they finally realized they
were dealing with somebody whose mind was made up. This is the
way I have to go. I think they've finally accepted that.

I've done a lot of research and talked to a lot of people who
have had success in treating cancer with alternative programs. I'm
going to do this and see what happens. And I'm trying to have a lot

of faith. Sometimes I talk to God. I say, Okay, this whole body is yours, including the tumor. You can take that away if you want to. I don't know what you want from me in this world, Lord, but I've done the best I could all through my life. I don't want it to end now.

I would say my husband is more stressed with what he's going through right now than he's ever been in his life. He runs errands to all the places I can't go. He represents us in battles with the insurance company for things we've lost, and is trying not to lose more. He works long hours, does all the work around the house and yard that I can't do, and goes to MCS support group meetings even when I can't go. He's the one who dragged me to a support group meeting when my brain was so dysfunctional that I didn't know what was going on, probably because somebody told him it would be good for us. He just said, "You're going!" I sat there like a zombie. People have told me that I just stared into space at the first few meetings I went to.

This has been very difficult on our marriage. Ron has had to make a lot of changes in his life in order to live in the same house with me. He's really going above and beyond. When he comes home from anyplace he has to take off his clothes, zip them into a garment bag until he can air them out on the weekend, take a shower and wash his hair even when he's exhausted. It's very emotionally draining. Sometimes when he wants to be close or give me a hug, I react to something he's picked up on his clothes from some place he's been. I'm telling him, "Get away! You're not safe! My mouth is burning!" And at the same time I'm telling him I need him and want to be close. Can you imagine how that affects our intimacy? Or, he'll bring in bags of groceries and I'll say, "There's something wrong with the grocery bags! Get them out of here!"

The isolation is tough, too. I've had to tell my family that I can't go visit them right now, so that I can get strong enough to be with them in the future. Some family members have triple washed their clothes in baking soda in an attempt to be safe for me. My dad is the only one, besides my husband, who has been able to make himself chemically free enough to be able to hug me safely. I write letters and talk on the telephone. And when I have been in isolation for so long that I think I can't stand it anymore, Ron and I try something to be a part of a group. But then I am usually deathly ill and unable to function the next day. So we go back into isolation until I get so lonely that I try again. A few weeks ago I wanted to go to church because

I've been too sick to go for three years. Another friend with MCS went with us to an outdoor service, where they agreed to put some chairs away from other people for us. Ron and Lori stayed but I didn't last ten minutes. I was reacting to fertilizers on the lawn. I was so nauseated and dizzy, and my mouth burned so badly, that I could hardly make it from my chair to the car. That's how my life is now when I try to go out in the world.

Before all this happened my husband and I worked with youth at our church. I was somebody who loved the unlovable. I went to International Special Olympics with a girl whose mother couldn't go. I was a huggy person; I put my arm around people and gave them hugs. My attitude is that if there's a human being on this earth, they are here for a purpose and have special gifts they're supposed to use. Now I'm wondering how I can do this when I'm living this isolated life.

Ron tells me, "You're not isolated, Peggy. You're there for every phone call every time someone in the support group calls you. You'll always be remembered for the advice and counseling you've done over the telephone." I have helped several people through suicidal chemical reactions like the ones I went through.

When people call me for support I don't always know what to say. But I do know that sometimes when you're at the end of the road and you don't know where you're going to go or how you're going to cope, you should just wait—just give it a little more time.

Don Paladin
Bellingham, Washington

Don Paladin served in the Vietnam War in the Army Security Agency. When his military duty ended he returned to college with a desire to teach special education. Upon completion of his master's degree he moved into a new mobile home and began the teaching career of his dreams. Five years later he consulted a physician due to severe fatigue. Told by the physician that he was sensitive to formaldehyde, Don moved out of the mobile home, although the diagnosis seemed unbelievable to him at the time. For the next seven years he struggled to maintain his career and recover his health. Eventually his career ended due to the severity of his chemical sensitivities. Still a teacher at heart, Don is committed to educating others about environmental health issues, and he is committed to his own personal growth. He is an MCS support group leader in Bellingham, and the creator and manager of the Washington State MCS Network (WSMCSN@aol.com), an Internet web page featuring state resources for MCS-friendly doctors, lawyers, organizations, support, publications and web sites. Washington State MCS Network also provides an interactive network of people and groups connected by e-mail to share information.

My philosophy has always been that you learn from what you don't understand. Evolution comes from the darkness, not the light. So this has been a learning experience for me. The cup is half full for me. Always has been. Although I do have days when it's half empty.

One of the hardest things for me now is not having a job. I always enjoyed what I did and had that to look forward to. I've had chemical sensitivities for fifteen years now. I taught with it for twelve years. Toward the end I worked part-time. I had twenty years vested in the system, so I hung on.

To hold onto my job, I had no social life. I came home, made dinner, did whatever work I had to do, then slept and went to work. That was my whole life. I couldn't be around most people, I was so sensitive to fragrances and other chemicals. It got worse and worse. Basically, I became an isolate. I was weak and fatigued and gave everything I had to surviving at work. I lost connections with friends and family and life in general. But I did the best I could with what I had.

As long as I could control the environment in my classroom, I could manage. I was doing all kinds of things to maintain—shiatsu, acupuncture, diet. I did all the latest. But the thing I didn't have control over was the application of pesticides in the building. Finally, I couldn't handle it when they were using pesticides in the classroom. I reacted too severely. It just made me useless.

The major turning point in my hypersensitivity happened in '86

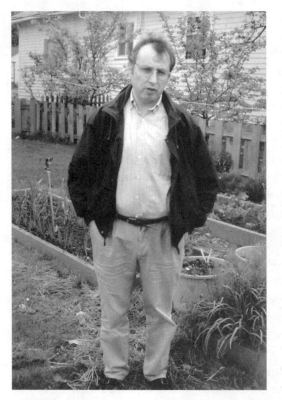

or '87, when I returned to my classroom in the fall. There was a wasp nest inside the fresh air exchange in my room. Pesticides were used to exterminate the wasps, despite the fact that I had made it known that I was chemically sensitive. Until that point I was still functioning pretty well.

I went into my classroom the afternoon after they had used the pesticides, and had the most horrendous experience of my life. Talk about visiting hell! I had panic attacks for a week, spasms and blurred vision. I couldn't function. I think I was off work for two weeks.

I really wanted to go back to teaching, but I couldn't go back into the classroom with the pesticides. So I finished that year teaching in a tiny little room, and I had a lot of health problems.

The next year they moved me to another room, after some negotiations. But there was diesel smoke coming into that room through the fresh air intake. One administrator was really supportive, but I think he basically got tired of going to bat for me. He encouraged me to take a disability leave. My doctor suggested I take a year off. I was trying to hold onto my job, and I thought I could get back to how I had felt earlier if I could just take a year off to build up my body. But the truth is, I never recovered my pre-pesticide-exposure health. I would say that I was forced out of my job because they were tired of dealing with me.

I always ask myself: Okay, what am I learning from this experience? I don't think we can go through life without learning from our negative experiences. Prior to my chemical sensitivity I used pesticides, herbicides, synthetics and all of that. I've learned so much in the past fifteen years about my body, the universe and ecology.

I've changed so much in my viewpoint on life and my way of interacting. When you have to live a very limited, controlled lifestyle, you find out what's really important.

There are days when I'm depressed and don't want to get out of bed. It would be easier to just close my eyes and sleep forever. When I have those negative periods I realize that, although I'm not comfortable in them, it's not the end, it's just a continuation of the day. So I persist and accept what I can do, and I listen to my body. If my body says I'm tired, I rest. I learned a long time ago to be respectful of my body. It always treats me much better that way.

Right now the most important thing to me is trying to create an oasis where I can function in a toxic world. I feel I need to use my limited energy to do something productive. I'm involved with a cohousing group, and we're planning to build an ecologically oriented small community here in the Bellingham area. Because they are ecologically minded people, they understand the consequences of adding poison to your environment. The main facilitator of the program plans to use nontoxic or low toxic construction materials. His wife is mildly chemically sensitive.

My hope is that we can create a model of sustainable housing. I want to create an alternative to what already exists. That's what I have to do to survive.

Although I think those of us with MCS need to work together, I really think cooperating with non–chemically injured people is probably what is going to work best for us. I would say having friends who are not chemically sensitive is probably more powerful in terms of encouragement. Those of us who are chemically sensitive don't always have the energy to encourage our peers. We can listen to each other, but we don't always have the dynamic productive energy that it takes to make things happen. Many are suffering from low self-esteem from the chemical injury, and feel disenfranchised, disempowered. We're just consumed with trying to deal with our own survival issues, whether it's being paid by Labor and Industry or trying to find solutions to our health problems.

There are people in the Washington Toxics Coalition—which I'm a member of—who aren't chemically injured but who are really supportive of us and advocate for us.

My biggest concern is that I'll become destitute—my pension will be gone or I'll become so debilitated because of exposures to pesticides that I can't function. But I realize that I've been really fortunate.

See, I was in Vietnam as a soldier, so I've visited a space where the possibility of extinction existed—personal extinction. You begin to realize that the most horrendous things aren't as bad as they appear, once you are experiencing them. When it rains, you protect yourself as best as you can from the elements, and wait till the sun comes back out.

That's kind of how I deal with fear, you know. I just remind myself that it's not permanent, and do some self-talking.

I'm not an angry person. Mostly, I get discouraged rather than angry. The hardest part for me as a teacher is not being able to make people understand the impact of low-level chemical exposures.

If people understand a problem, there can be resolution to the problem. People just don't understand unless it affects them personally to the same degree. MCS is hard to understand even when you have it.

In '85 I visited a woman in California who was sensitive. The whole trip was horrendous, I was reacting to so many things. But I remember that she was driving a little Honda and she had sealed all the air vents. I thought, oh come on—you can't be *that* sensitive!

That has really come around to haunt me because, now, ten years later, I'm doing the same thing because I have the same problem. After the pesticide exposure in the school I was so sensitive I had to seal the car because driving just a few blocks bothered me. Then I became sensitive to the air conditioning, perfumes, you name it. Hopefully I'm getting that out of my system now that I'm avoiding chemicals and following an organic diet to lighten my load. I'm not as sensitive as I was. Last fall friends would come over and I could smell the soap they washed their skin with.

By sharing my story I hope to help other people understand, have someone say, "Aha! That touches what I understand!" For me, that's what life has been about as a teacher and as a human being, helping people understand, making connections, helping those synapses to fire in the brain.

I really believe this is about personal empowerment. It's important for people with chemical sensitivities to say, "I don't have psychological problems. These products are poisonous and just because you don't understand that doesn't make it not so." All of us on this planet are entitled to be in a space where we are not poisoned or injured by others' reckless behavior.

The solution comes from each of us finding answers and creating understanding for ourselves. It's important for our self-esteem to *do* something. In my support group I try to encourage others to find and understand information and to help others. It's mostly about giving people power and information to give *other* people power and information.

I believe in personal evolution. I don't ever look at where I'm at as being a final point, I see it as growth and personal evolution.

We're all kind of entwined in this evolution that we're going through. The whole planet is out of balance right now, and we who have chemical sensitivities are suffering the consequences of that. And I don't think it's just those of us with chemical sensitivities, it's people with cancer and other illnesses created by our toxic environment.

The message being sent to the dominant culture right now is that you can't use poisons without a consequence. We *are* that message. I think our whole planet is going to make some major shifts and changes in a positive way. In whatever way we can create a loving, nurturing, caring environment, we will flourish.

Jill Holden
Seattle, Washington

A local massage clinic made an appointment for me to see Jill Holden when I requested a licensed massage practitioner that would be completely unscented. A native of Madison, Wisconsin, Jill, thirty-one when interviewed, has a bachelor's degree in theater, and enjoys hiking, reading, journaling, and learning about herbs. As a volunteer she teaches adults to read.

Multiple chemical sensitivity has shaped Jill's life, but is not a significant part of her self-image. Although the symptoms she experiences from chemical exposures can be debilitating, she does not think of herself as handicapped or sick, nor does she seek out friendship or support from others with MCS.

After she realized that she had MCS, Jill discovered she had breast cancer. That discovery was a catalyst in her journey toward wellness that led to her new and liberating lifestyle.

As an adolescent I started developing ear infections and sinusitis. When I was about fifteen I started developing eczema. Back then I was being treated by allopathic doctors who were treating me with antibiotics.

After I graduated from college in Green Bay I moved to Chicago, in '82, and worked in professional theater—a really toxic world. I was around nasty chemicals all the time, like dry-cleaning fluid, acetone, all that stuff. I never wore a mask or anything. I just cringe about that now, thinking what that was doing to my liver and body. But at that point it either didn't bother me or I wasn't aware of it because my body was so polluted that I didn't know the difference.

When I got to Seattle, in '93, I was pretty sick. I had hives all over my body and eczema all over my hands. It was painful, especially in massage school where my hands were in contact with water all the time. They used to hurt so bad that I had to keep socks on them, and when I was waitressing I'd have to get people to wipe the tables for me. If I put rubber gloves on I reacted to the rubber. Before I knew any better, I was using cortisone and lost a layer of skin on my hands.

Before I knew I was chemically sensitive I began to notice the smells from bleaches and cleaners in the grocery store. I cannot go down that aisle.

When I finally went to a naturopath, that's when the pieces of the puzzle finally started coming together. I realized, yes, I did indeed have allergies. I had many, many food allergies that were never detected, and taking all those antibiotics had set me up for candida to grow and it weakened my immune system.

A lot of people don't have the resources that we have in this part of the country. Here there are a lot of naturopathic practitioners and people who are more aware of environmental health issues. We're in the hub of it, and I start thinking that's the way it is for everybody. But that's not true. There are some places where it's polluted and no one understands. That's got to be very hard and isolating when nobody takes you seriously.

In the beginning of all this I thought, poor me, my life is over. It took me a while to get through that. The first year was really hard for me because I was grieving. I thought, I can't eat bread, I can't eat fruit, I can't, I can't, I can't! Then I started learning more about my body, and herbs, and acupuncture and that type of thing. I started feeling more empowered. I started getting rid of anything in my house that wasn't natural.

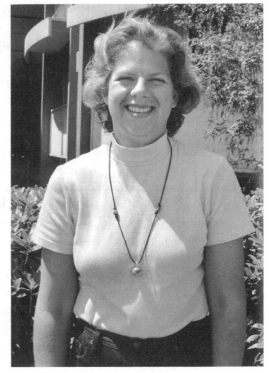

Then, last year, I discovered I had a fibrous growth in my breast about four or five inches long. And it grew very rapidly. I didn't want to have it removed, but I finally agreed to. I thought that was the end of it, but when a biopsy was done there were cancer cells found inside it. It was a cancer that rarely will metastasize, and when it does it goes to the chest, so it's contained; it is not genetically linked. As far as cancers go, this is not a bad one to have. But it does not respond to chemotherapy or radiation.

I could have just curled up in a ball and thought, I've got cancer, I'm going to do whatever the doctors tell me, or, I'm not going to get out of bed. Or, I could do what I did. I took charge. I knew I wasn't going to die, that this was not life threatening. But I knew it was a life-altering thing. I had five weeks before they were going to do another surgery, a partial mastectomy, and I was just dreading this. I was very proactive in my treatment and in my healthcare. I thought: this is my body, my time, and my money. I brought questions with me and I took notes. I kept telling myself positive things and used visualization. I'd lay down on the ground and do relaxation techniques and visualize my tumor shrinking. I really tried to keep a good attitude and stay connected with myself. I had a great surgeon who was open to alternative medicine and healing of the mind.

Before that, I had a doctor who wasn't like that, so I just didn't go back to him.

I like to think of myself as somebody who's kind of carefree and spontaneous, but, in reality, I prepare physically and mentally for situations in my life, especially if I know they're going to be a challenge. I just saw the cancer as another challenge. I don't think I could have done that if the cancer had happened two years earlier, when I first started dealing with my allergies. It would have been too overwhelming. My attitude has completely changed since then.

I was preparing physically and mentally for the second surgery. I got my body into shape like I was training to be in a marathon. I exercised every day, and my endorphins were going, and I was feeling good. I was really happy. I had never really exercised that much. I started jogging and swimming, and I joined a gym.

I also started looking closer at everything in my house and got rid of a lot more things that I had thought were natural but really weren't. I started reading the labels and seeing all these chemicals. I just cleaned everything out. That was empowering! When you do things for yourself it has a psychological benefit. To say, I don't need all this stuff, made me feel better. I opened up my cupboard and thought, I don't need any of this stuff, and got rid of it. That, for me, was so cool to simplify my life like that. I just love it.

I cleaned house physically and spiritually. I thought more about my life. I consider myself a seeker now. I'm on a spiritual quest. I don't adhere to any organized religion, but I feel a connection with people, the universe, the earth. I'm still trying to figure it all out for myself. Spirituality helps me to see the bigger picture. Keeping the proper attitude was, and still is, essential to my healthcare—keeping that sense of being alive, a sense of joy, and connecting with the earth and people. I can choose to die or I can choose to live. I think I have a lot of say in that.

With my first surgery I was really tired and I had a lot of inflammation and I took some painkillers. After the second surgery I healed so much quicker, and I took absolutely no painkillers. Physically, I lost part of my body. But, at the same time I felt alive and liberated and good. I had this kind of transformation.

As far as I know the cancer is gone. It was just something that happened. A lot of fibrous breast tissue is related to poor liver function. I can't be sure if there was a direct correlation, but I know the more cleaning out I do and the more cleansing, the better for me.

I don't consider my chemical sensitivities debilitating. They're annoying. I get brain fog and headaches, and I think they affect me hormonally and emotionally. It's hard to tell if I'm angry and resentful because people are wearing fragrances or because the fragrances affect my emotions. I know other people aren't trying to hurt me, so I have to find a tactful way of letting them know what's bothering me. How I present myself affects how seriously people take me. I worked with another woman who was more sensitive than I was, and she expressed herself differently than I do. She came off as whiny, not someone who is proactive, so she was not taken as seriously as I was. I don't know if I've alienated anyone, but sometimes I think I'm willing to pay that price for my health if it's something really hurting me. That's taking responsibility for me.

My reactions are not sudden, they're more subtle. So I sometimes ignore a fragrance when it first hits me, thinking that maybe I'll be okay. I just try to act normal. But then I get hit with a delayed reaction.

It's hard when I have a reaction when I'm giving a massage because I'm touching the person and holding my head away from them at the same time, and I can taste the chemicals in my mouth. If someone comes in who's a smoker, it effervesces through their skin into mine. It's horrible. I've said, "I'm really sorry, but this isn't working and you're not going to get quality treatment." I try to be as nice as I can. I can't just blurt it out because it might come from an angry place if I do. I have to make sure that I'm thinking clearly, which is hard because I can't think clearly when I'm exposed to a fragrance.

I've found that if I bring in coffee beans, put them in a little cup, and snort it, I can clear my sinuses and nasal passages. I also carry lavender with me because lavender clears the air. If there's a smell that's hard for me, I smell the coffee beans or put a little lavender on my temples to try to change the air. And I tell people that we have a fragrance-free policy.

Most people are really understanding. They say, "Oh, I'm sorry! I didn't know." But my former boss, of all people, came in wearing perfume from time to time. One day I said, "I want to tell you something, but I don't want you to get upset. I need to let you know that I'm very allergic to perfume, and it's hard for me to work because perfume makes my heart palpitate and I feel dizzy." It hurt me because she knows me really well, and knows I'm chemically sensitive, and we had a fragrance-free policy there.

I don't get hit with it every day, especially in the kind of environment I'm in with a lot of people who are very health conscious and don't wear a lot of perfume. I know I'm sensitive, but I forget about it a lot. For me, it's not the number one issue. I usually don't think about it until something happens. It can be something like someone switching deodorants.

I love body work. Massage is my job and it's my passion. And, I've really been getting interested in herbs. I'm thinking about taking a class or doing an apprenticeship. I'd like to learn how to cultivate herbs and make my own tinctures. That's been really exciting for me.

I work out every day now and, if I can get in a walk, too, I'll do that. That saved me last winter from seasonal affective disorder. I get affected by the weather and by hormones. I'm pretty good at identifying it now, and I can shake myself out of it. I know it's really good for me to be social when it happens. I'll call a friend and say, "Let's go to Buddha class"—that's a meditation class.

I love to go hiking and camping, to be outdoors. I like to write in my journal and read. I have a lot of friends. And I do volunteer work for the Literacy Action Council, to teach people how to read—it's a one-on-one thing. I've always wanted to do that, to do something different than massage as a volunteer, and I always enjoyed English.

I don't know if I want a cure for chemical sensitivities. This stuff isn't good for people and it's not good for our environment. We don't need all these products. Once I stopped using all the stuff I thought I needed, my body did fine without it. I don't need to use soap. Apple cider vinegar or lemon juice works for deodorant, and lemon juice works as hairspray and gives your hair highlights. I usually use baking soda to clean my teeth, and a lot of flossing. I don't use any cleaning products in my apartment except vinegar and baking soda.

My roommate and I had to work through a conflict. Her boyfriend sent her this French perfume and she was going into her room and putting a little bit on, thinking that much wouldn't hurt me. But I could smell it a mile away. The whole place smelled and made me sick. It was a real issue for a while until one day I said, "If I were to go into anaphylactic shock, would you be spraying perfume?" She said no and agreed not to wear it anymore. It's really hard for people who've never been chemically sensitive to understand that it's not personal, it's real, and there are different effects.

I think people who are chemically sensitive are like the frogs that are growing three legs and the alligators that are changing sexes. These are all indications that there are a lot of toxins and environmental poisons that our bodies cannot handle. The chemicals in our environment aren't good for anybody.

Christina Jacobs
Portland, Oregon

Fears of homelessness lie dormant in most people, until health or resources are in jeopardy. Any catastrophic or chronic illness can bring those fears and the possibility of homelessness closer to the surface. People with MCS and electromagnetic fields sensitivity (EMFS) are particularly vulnerable. Christina Jacobs is one example, and a model for facing the reality of homelessness with hope and perseverance. She has lived out of her car for most of seven years.

Christina believes that each time someone goes through a difficult period and emerges with priceless wisdom and increased inner strength, we all benefit in some way. If this is true—and I believe it is—then the world is a better place for her presence. Her story is one that can arouse deep fear, open you to your own inner strength, or both. It is a story of desperation, not easy to read.

A native of Portland, Christina is a former world-class athlete and former massage therapist with a B.A. in Russian and Japanese languages, now working toward a doctorate in naturopathic medicine. Hoping to eventually receive grants to pay for her education, she currently pays for classes with a part of her monthly disability income of several hundred dollars.

I was given Christina's name and voice mail number from a friend of hers in Santa Fe. When I made contact with her in Oregon, she was planning a trip to Washington. She came with her dog Luna to my home for the interview and to spend the night. Part coyote and part guardian angel, Luna is a loving and loyal companion to Christina.

Articulate, intelligent and deep, Christina moved me beyond the stereotypes of homelessness to a greater trust in my own ability to cope under any circumstances. Some of the statements in the following narrative were written by her on applications she made to medical school and for grants. I included these because I feel they express who she is so beautifully.

Christina chose to use a pseudonym for this narrative, to protect her privacy.

The number of people who are homeless due to MCS and EMFS is unknown.

I'm a human being with strong points and weak points just like everybody else. Sometimes I feel like I'm a cross between a homeless person and a camper, but I don't have a stove or any frills. I have experienced great extremes in my life and have developed a deep level of human understanding and compassion.

In my teen years I captured the world record in the marathon. I was one of the first American women to attain this honor. My world record run was an inspiration to many and was the trigger event that brought women's marathon running into the United States. It was rewarding to be influential in creating changes to bring respect and opportunity for women and girls in long-distance running.

I was one of six runners who qualified to compete in Europe where I placed ninth in the world. I won six biathlon championships and several triathlon championships. My running coach was Steve Prefontaine, and that is one of my most cherished experiences as an athlete. I also had the honor of serving as a massage therapist to Olympic- and national-class athletes, and establishing an athletic program to assist them in their training. I am familiar with humans expressing their exceptional physical strength.

I have some shame about my lifestyle now. For most of the past seven years I've lived in my car because I'm disabled from sensitivities to chemicals and electromagnetic fields (EMFs), and because of my financial situation. I don't like to use the word disability, because I have hope that I won't always be this way.

If I had more money I could create a safe living space for myself, and I'm certain that would make me feel a little more grounded to the planet. Sometimes I'm a little worried for myself now that I've been in the car so long. The lack of connection to society is starting to tip the balance. I can feel my feet barely touching the earth at times, like I'm barely here anymore. But I do have an inner strength. Of the choices available to me with my means, I'm still choosing the one that's most nurturing and potentially the most life transforming to me. Knowing that, it makes sense to me to live the way I do for now. It's just not what other people are doing.

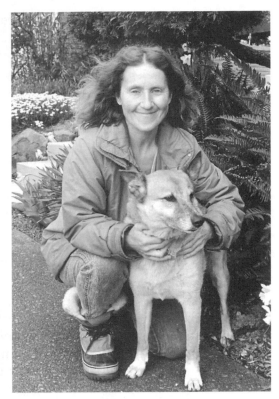

My willingness to check very deeply within my heart and soul to find the truth and to follow it, even in extremely chaotic or painful situations, is the essence of my strength. That's what I have. That's my core. It's a bit similar to when I was a long-distance runner. The discipline acquired through marathon training has prepared me to overcome emotional, physical and professional challenges.

A couple times in races everyone was so far ahead of me that I'd think, did I jump into the wrong race or something? But if I could focus deep inside myself, acknowledge that I was last, do everything I could to make a little change for myself—which in running terms would be to check my arm movement and my breathing—then I had a pretty strong ability to tune out everything else and just be me. That would have a great impact on my ability to move up in the race, and often finish in first place despite my slow beginning. That skill now helps to sustain me.

After college I created a pretty nice lifestyle for myself, working as a massage therapist and competing in triathlons. In 1988 a traumatic injury to my back resulted in serious immune and nervous system complications. I think that may have been a part of what made me susceptible to chemical sensitivities. I quickly changed from being very active to being physically crippled. I still swam a little because that's one of the only exercises you can do with a back injury, but I was getting sicker and sicker. Soon the chlorine began to cause spasms in my feet, so I had to stop swimming. My joints ached, my sense of smell increased. In a pretty short period of time my health deteriorated so badly that I had to crawl because I couldn't walk, and was able to sit for only a few minutes at a time. I had to crawl to the front door to let the dogs out. Muscles in my legs would tear just from turning my head while lying in bed. Sometimes my skin would split and tear. For six months, I felt I was on the edge of death.

Many of my running friends seemed frightened when they saw my body going through these changes, and turned away. My family is also frightened by crisis situations. Except for my nephews, my family has been unable to comprehend my physical and emotional challenges. I believe they feel shame because I don't have a "normal" life. I don't fit in. I think they believe that if I would just act a little more normal our family would be "okay." Though I have received some financial support from my family, it has been given without an understanding of my very painful and urgent circumstances. I actually feel more homeless when I stay near my family than I do when I'm on the road. I do derive a great deal of satisfaction from my relationships with my nephews, and it feels important to me to stay involved in their lives. It's probably scary for them to see their aunt in trouble, and in pain. When I first suffered my back injury we shifted our activities from going for a run to things like watching movies or baking cookies together.

It isn't just my family. I'm an eyesore to most people. I think my lifestyle is frightening to others because they are afraid it could happen to them. There are some people who can really see inside other people. They can still see you even if you can live in a car or have some other funny lifestyle. There aren't that many people who are that pure. Even in a seminar where people are willing to look deeper to see others for who they really are, I can stick out pretty easily. It isn't difficult for people to figure out I'm living in my car. It's a little too much. It makes people feel uncomfortable.

There are some people who would look at my situation and think my health problems were the result of a post-traumatic stress disorder, or depression or both. As a child I was abused, and nearly died from anorexia before the age of ten.

I would agree that childhood trauma could have made me more susceptible to any disease. But people would be missing critical pieces of the picture if they didn't also factor in the physical and biochemical aspects. An unhealthy environment also affects people who don't have a history of abuse or family problems. And, in cases like mine where there might be a psychosocial connection, that doesn't mean the MCS is any less real.

When I was so sick that I was crawling, there wasn't anyone to help me. Mold was growing in my dirty dishes from sitting in the sink so long. I was desperate to find a way to gather back some health, and my willpower from running sustained me as I went from doctor to doctor.

The first doctor to finally help diagnosed me with mercury poisoning. That gave me hope. I made an appointment to have my amalgams removed at a clinic in Colorado Springs, but I had to wait two or three months. I didn't know if I would live that long. I thought, well, maybe I'll be here and maybe I won't. I was so sick I could hardly move, but it helped me to have a focus. I really struggled to not die.

One doctor told me, "It's very hard to poison an athlete, but once you do it's actually easier because an athlete's whole body system is set up to facilitate blood supply." He thought that might be why I became so debilitated after my injury.

After my amalgams were removed I was bounding up and down stairs and had a life again. Two months later I had bridges put in my mouth and my health deteriorated a second time. Before long I was back to being crippled. The dentist who did the bridge work had promised to test my compatibility to different materials. When I started feeling worse again I asked him to double check that he had used only materials that I was compatible with. He wrote a letter to me saying that everything checked out fine. A year later I finally had the bridges removed because I knew they were making me sick, I didn't care what anyone said. Then I had the materials tested and found that the dentist had lied to me. He later admitted he had not used the dental materials he told me he had used. He had taken advantage of me by claiming to be a holistic physician.

The next step was to have some crowns put on my teeth. Shortly after that work was finished I went to stay with some friends. They had just installed a new floor in their home, and I reacted to the glue. I became so ill I could hardly walk. After that, I started reacting to everything in my environment. When you're that sick there is a fine line between what is helpful and what is too much. Even Reiki was more than I could handle.

I had just rented a little house where they were going to do some renovations, so I asked them to use nontoxic paints and sealers, and I paid the difference. I learned that a good sleep in a nontoxic environment is essential to healing, so I bought a cotton futon and put my focus on creating a good sleeping space. I lived in only one room in the house and kept the doors and windows wide open all the time. But my reactions continued to be so severe that I started staying outdoors most of the time, just trying to survive. My ability to sleep and to tolerate chemical exposures improved when I quit trying to sleep in the house. That's one of the main reasons I live out of my car. Out in the natural elements, in pure darkness and away from electromagnetic influences, I sleep like a baby. What I didn't understand then was that it was the beginning of something that would last a long time. But I didn't really have a choice. Finally I stopped looking for a safe place to live because it seemed like it would take nothing short of a miracle.

It's a struggle to be on the road and feel like there's no safe place for me on the planet. Sometimes I drive an hour and a half to find a good place to park. Good sleep is so important to recovering my health that I probably am a little more willing than the average person to go to extremes to get that. And it has paid off. Today I can hike and I can sit for normal periods.

A doctor in Santa Fe strengthened my nervous system and stabilized my condition and later provided me with the opportunity to assist him for a while. It was a temporary situation that met some of my needs at that time. When my health was more stable I came back to Portland, but I was still unable to work. My sensitivity to electromagnetics had not improved significantly. Fluorescent lights, telephones, power lines and fuse boxes are the things that really affect me the most. After prolonged exposures I can have difficulty finding my way on the road, my heart beats irregularly, and I develop insomnia. It affects my brain and is very disorienting. Massage work is so strenuous it no longer is a viable option for me.

Through my experiences with the doctor I worked with and my own healing journey I was exposed to cutting-edge medical techniques, and was inspired to return to school to obtain a naturopathic doctorate degree. Over the last four years I have completed thirty-five courses on health-related topics. In 1998 I was accepted into the naturopathic doctorate program at the University of Natural Medicine in Santa Fe, and awarded seventy credit hours toward my degree for my previous course work and experience. The curriculum is offered almost exclusively as an independent study program, which enables me to live and study off campus. In a regular classroom, the use of fluorescent lights alone would exclude me from participation.

If the wisdom and insight gained from all of my experiences can help to make even one person's life a little easier, or can facilitate even one person to become aware of his or her ability to heal from within, then my endeavor to become a naturopathic physician is worthwhile to me. Once I am established in my practice, I want to donate some percentage of my time to providing service and treatment to people who have become isolated or disenfranchised from friends, family or society due to injury, illness, prejudice, abuse, or because they are compassionate human beings living in a fast-moving society.

I never would have survived my debilitating injury and illness without the gracious help of fine physicians. I look forward to one day passing on to others some of the wisdom, compassion and medical interventions that have been so helpful to me. Hopefully I can help others with chemical and electromagnetic sensitivities to overcome their fears and to strengthen their bodies so that their tolerance can be increased.

Besides a medical degree I also hope to achieve other goals that are important to me. One day I'd like to have a piece of land, and buy or build a little house in the wilderness—maybe a straw-bale house—have a deck, or a living room with big windows, where I could locate my bed to be close to the moon at night. I also hope to find a special man to love and marry, and to have a family. I've spent a lot of time with children, as an aunt and as a nanny, and I enjoy the kind of unconditional love that children can express so easily.

In the meantime, I'm paying for medical school out of my disability checks. That seems like a stupid thing to do when I'm dealing with core survival, too hungry at times to think straight. I don't always know where I'm going to get my next meal. But I don't see how I can get out of the trap I'm in without taking steps toward moving beyond survival. Working toward this goal enables me to see a spark of hope. I've applied for services with vocational rehabilitation. If I received some assistance from them, maybe then I wouldn't have to pay for classes with my disability income. If I used all of my money for food and basic needs I might see another shift in my health. I need help to get out of the place I'm in.

Survival takes up a lot of time and energy. I'm in survival mode more than most people, figuring out what to eat when I can. Sometimes I crave eating three meals a day and not worrying about my next meal. Although I have food sensitivities, it's sometimes more important that I eat whatever I can, even if it's not the best foods for me. I try to eat high-quality organic food whenever possible. When I eat good organic food and flax seed oil, then I have more tolerance for a while. I wouldn't eat real junk foods, because that's not real food anyway.

Another difficulty is finding a bathroom to use. I use restrooms in grocery and health food stores, but I'm not comfortable going to the same place on a regular basis. I feel like I'm developing digestive problems from not releasing when I need to.

Laundering my clothes and linens is another challenge. Sometimes I drive two hours to Eugene to do my laundry because there is a smoke-free laundromat and it is a city where there is more tolerance for people with alternative lifestyles.

In Florida I was asked to leave campgrounds where I'd paid the fees, and I've been told by a police officer that he would have to arrest me if I was living in my car. But one time in Arizona a woman came up to me and asked if I was living in my car. That's not an easy question for me, and I'm not particularly friendly if I'm asked by someone I don't know because of my experiences. But this woman said, "I lived in my car for a while and I had the most wonderful time of my life." She looked like a normal, healthy woman, and well-dressed. I don't know what her story was. If I'd been friendlier she probably would have told me. Maybe she had been camping, and had the resources to protect herself. But it was nice to see this woman and to hear her appreciation for the positive benefits of my current way of life.

In terms of my personal safety, I've been lucky. I've been "assaulted" by people's disapproving looks, and by chemical and electromagnetic exposures I didn't detect when I parked my car at night. But that's different from someone coming at me. I have to strike a balance by finding an environmentally safe place to sleep without it being too isolated, where I'm more vulnerable. My goal is to sleep soundly, so I have to feel as safe as possible. I have my dog with me, and she gives me a sense of safety. And I'm also careful about staking out the area. I've learned that I will wake up if there's something really wrong, and that I can trust that on a deep level. When that happens I don't question it at the time, because coming from a deep sleep I might not be thinking clearly. I just wake up and drive off immediately. I park my car in position to drive off quickly if necessary.

There's certainly no glory in being homeless. But I know the country and the earth's cycles better than most people. I've had a chance to run into a black bear in the woods. And I've really connected to the sun and the moon. I know other people can see the moon at night, but it's really different when the moon is shining on your face. It's really quite healing. When I'm sleeping in my car, I feel safe knowing that the moon is right there. I probably know how to make something out of nothing, and how to survive better than the average person. And I can see in the dark.

I've had incredible experiences with life. It's sad and lonely and sometimes I wonder if there's a place in the world for someone like me. But I have an inner strength from my training as a world-class runner. Sometimes I wanted to win a race so bad, and I started out last. I often ended up in first place. And the reality is that I'm living in my car. But when I look at people who are living unconsciously, and who don't seem to have a deep level of compassion, I've wondered: Who is more alive—them or me?

Robbynne Martin
Seattle, Washington

When I first met Robbynne Martin it never occurred to me that she would be a subject for this book. Assisting a health care professional I saw for treatments, she looked radiantly well. Sometimes she was the one to apply pressure to my ankles, wrists, neck and arms to facilitate the acupressure treatment process. I looked forward to her gentle touch and healing spirit, and was surprised to learn that for a twelve-year period she had been deathly ill and severely chemically sensitive.

Robbynne's MCS began in her early thirties when she was working in a prefabricated classroom that was off-gassing formaldehyde. Then, the sudden deaths of both her brother and her husband contributed further to a downward spiral of her physical and mental health, and she became completely disabled. Equally dramatic is the story of her recovery, a long, slow process of medical interventions and spiritual awakenings. The focus of this interview is on the spiritual aspects of her recovery, which she believes were instrumental in the success of her medical treatments. Some people might find parts of her story difficult to believe, particularly those events which she describes as "woo-woo" experiences. Some might reject her perspective on the mind-body-spirit connection, or incorrectly assume she views depression or mental illness as the cause of MCS. Robbynne attributes her chemical sensitivity to a chemical overload, a genetic predisposition, and the physical burden of emotional trauma.

As a child raised on a dairy farm on Puget Sound, she developed asthma and allergies, including a severe allergy to milk. Undiagnosed for several years, the milk allergy resulted in frequent infections and tonsillitis so severe that her hearing and speech were severely impaired. Through surgery her hearing returned to normal, and her speech was corrected with therapy.

Despite poor health as a child Robbynne developed a strong and independent spirit. After high school she immersed herself in other cultures in the U.S. and abroad before finally earning a degree as a teacher and reading specialist in Madison, Wisconsin. Many years into her process of recovery from MCS she earned a master's degree in transpersonal psychology. She wrote her dissertation on "Healing Through Grace: Cultivating the Receptive Heart."

When I met Robbynne she was about to move out of state to a warmer climate. The interview took place in her home in the Ananda Community, a spiritually based cohousing group in the Seattle area.

Healing isn't always dramatic. It can take a long while. And there is all this fear in the meantime. I've learned to keep my fear at bay by holding a receptive heart, keeping my boundaries close, and hanging onto God for dear life. If it hadn't been for the spiritual experiences I've had, I don't think I'd be alive today.

Most people have a bit of chemical sensitivity. So, in the general population I'm now average. I used to sit way out there at the very sensitive end. I'm so much better now I can handle almost anything. But I still use air cleaners and I'm not going to stay in a toxic environment or eat toxic food just because I can handle it. Some things just aren't good for people and it is best to avoid them. And I know there are chemicals that still can make me sick. The other day I collapsed in a dental chair when I reacted to an injection. I wasn't expecting that.

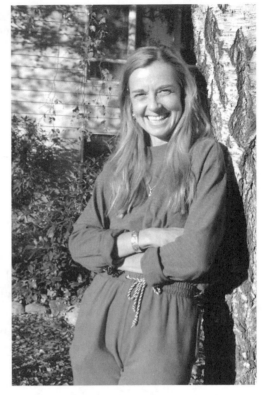

I was always known for being a buoyant, cheerful person, and independent. In my early thirties smells started getting to me. It started with the smell of glue and formaldehyde in these prefabricated rooms where I worked as a counselor. We also had an old Victorian house where we had redone every inch of it using every kind of chemical and solvent you could use. So I was around all of those chemicals, too. I suddenly began to notice diesel fumes, bathroom air fresheners and fabric softeners, things that had never bothered me before. At first it was just annoying, it was so strong. Then, one day I went to a little mall where they were changing the carpet. My eyes stung and swelled up, my asthma flared and my head started to hurt. The smell of the glue made me feel like I was going crazy and I ran outside. I'd never had an experience like that before.

After that I started reacting to potpourri and all kinds of fragrances. I absolutely could not go into shops with scents. Later the headaches got worse and I began to notice a little tremor in my brain. I still hadn't yet reached the point where I would lose my thoughts completely. I was able to continue teaching but I had to cut back to part-time, because my body was letting me know that it needed rest.

That was a difficult period of my life. My brother was killed by an intruder in his home, which caused a shock to my system. It threw me into a lot of mortality issues and I became depressed and fearful. I was able to take an antidepressant which worked wonderfully for me.

Another difficulty facing me at that time was an ethical crisis at my job. I was beside myself, not knowing how to handle the situation. Every time I tried to speak up at work, I was told by the administrators to keep quiet. I was getting more and more uncomfortable about it.

A friend suggested that I go to see some women who practiced Reiki in a church. I had not been practicing anything spiritual at all for fourteen years. I hadn't even been in a church. But when I went that evening I had a sudden spiritual awakening.

The second the two Reiki practitioners touched me, I felt like my body started spinning. I felt like I was spinning so fast that I might vomit. I don't remember anything else about the next forty-five minutes of the treatment. When it was over I sensed that I was different, but I didn't yet know how.

I went home from that session and went out for a walk. It was a beautiful spring day and still light outside. Suddenly the roses and the flower gardens and the trees all shimmered. People were shimmering. I had this incredibly intense joy, and I had this buzzing going on at the top of my head. I was filled with a sense of oneness with everything. It was strange. Everything was so alive and so intense that I hardly knew how to cope with it, to tell you the truth.

While I was out walking I prayed about my situation at work. I told God that I still didn't know how to deal with this ethical crisis. All of a sudden I felt Christ's presence and heard the message, "You must answer to the highest within you." In that moment I understood that we're all merged, we're all a part of this incredible thing called God. This was a very profound experience for me.

Shortly after that my husband and I sold our house and moved back to the Northwest. We moved into an old house and re-did parts of it. I was pretty careful about the products we used but things still bothered me a lot. There was more pollution here and my chemical illness worsened.

Two years later my husband died unexpectedly, and my world was blown apart again. I felt scared and angry because I was left alone in the world just when we were starting to think about having children. It was a few days before I turned thirty-five. It was such a shock that I couldn't sleep for months. My immune system crashed from the grief and sorrow. My red and white blood counts went way down. Epstein-Barr virus showed up. My spleen swelled and hurt all the time. I was diagnosed with post-traumatic stress disorder.

The trauma of his death had such an impact on me physically that I couldn't tolerate things that hadn't bothered me before. I was so vulnerable and shocked that my body just shut down. I reacted to everything I ate and everything in my environment. I tried to take an antidepressant, the same one that worked for me earlier. It sent zinging feelings all through my legs. The nerve endings in my legs were so painful at night that I couldn't move. I couldn't tolerate any anti-depressants at all.

During that period I also had a severe reaction to mercury from some dental work I had done. I was so horribly sick that I really thought I might die. Another time I thought I might die when I reacted to a medication with seizure activity for twenty-four hours. All I could do was sit in a rocking chair to wait it out.

I tried to go back to teaching half-time, but didn't make it to the end of the year. When I was near an odor I felt weak, like I was going to faint. I'd be fine until a kid would lean over my desk and I'd get a whiff of cologne or fabric softener. That smell would go right to my brain, and then I couldn't put my words into order. I was getting tremors so bad they were like seizures. That's when I got the most frightened. Everywhere I went I wore a mask. During the worst of it I carried oxygen in my car.

My family was very supportive. Some of them thought I was eccentric and beyond normal grief. But I have other family members who have chemical sensitivities, so they were pretty understanding. They didn't think I should stay in my house after my husband died, and they were right. But I'm real independent, and I wouldn't leave. So family members took turns coming to my house to stay with me. I couldn't even talk to anyone, my nervous system was so shot. They would just come and sit and read and leave me alone.

One day I knew I needed to go to a hospital. I think it was a plea for a sense of groundedness and safety, because I thought I was losing touch with reality. I stayed there for about twelve days, but it was unbearable because I was reacting to everything I ate in the hospital and I wasn't getting the nurturing and safety I needed. So I left the hospital and lived with different relatives for a while, like a bag lady.

Then I knew I needed to live alone for a while in order to heal. For two years I couldn't even watch TV, my nervous system was so sensitive. About all I could cope with was sitting on the beach. Even a massage would open up more grief than I could handle. I did start to improve, but I was very sick and weak. Occasionally I went to a family gathering, and twice a week I had appointments with my doctor, a clinical ecologist. A lot of them were telephone appointments because I was too sick to go to his office. He was on call for me and pulled me through some very difficult times.

During that period I could see what was happening. I could see that when a shock like that goes through your system you have to let it surface slowly. I just had to go totally inward and trust being alone and letting the grief come out at its own pace.

My father became very concerned, and he took me to another hospital where I stayed for four or five days. I met a really good psychiatrist there who worked with me for a year or so after I left the hospital. He specialized in post-traumatic stress disorder.

When I left the hospital my father wanted me to live with him and my stepmother. They made the house nontoxic, and for three months they didn't talk to me unless I talked to them, because I couldn't handle the stimulation. My father rocked me on his lap at night while I cried myself to sleep. I didn't know it at that time, but he rocked me even though his back was in a lot of pain. He was really there for me. That was my lowest point, the months before and during the time I lived with my father. For a year and a half I'd been deathly ill and emotionally ill. It was three years after my husband's death. On the surface it looked like I was doing everything I should be doing, seeing counselors and doing everything right. But underneath it all, I really wanted to die.

That changed when I had what I call a "woo-woo" experience. I don't remember much about it except that I was given a choice and I made a decision to live. Then I had another profound spiritual experience, a real turning point for me. I don't know how to explain it. It was a combination of Christ's words and heart letting me know that my husband was okay and that I was forgiven for anything wrong I had ever done or ever would do. On some level I had felt responsible for my husband's death. That's what I'd been holding in. My physical health began to respond better to medical interventions when I began to forgive myself. I think that was because I stopped struggling against myself. Forgiveness is crucial. It's number one.

After that experience I knew that I was going to be okay, but I still had a long way to go. My immune system was still so weak that I sometimes felt like I was close to dying. I was so thin and weak that I had to take hot showers in the middle of the night, I felt so cold, even though the temperature in my bedroom was ninety degrees.

For months after that I worked on cleansing my body of toxins. One of the things I learned was that if you do physical cleansing and healing, you're going to also be doing emotional and spiritual cleansing and healing. Whether you think you are or not, it happens. There is no separation. Illness is about being out of balance physically, emotionally, spiritually.

I had a lot of anger work to do, and did a lot of it by writing in a journal. I became aware that some of my thoughts and feelings were toxic to me, too. For example, if I believe that I am selfish—which is a toxic thought—I'll create guilt about it, and guilt is a toxic reaction.

When I got stronger I moved back to my house and began doing volunteer work at a hospice. I continued to use my respirator and mask for three years, because my body was still quite sensitive. As I got stronger I allowed myself to eat more foods, a little bit at a time, in order to allow my body to slowly develop trust. I still lived reclusively because I felt overstimulated so easily. I needed that time alone to heal my nervous system.

I used to keep a meditation place in a closet with no clothes or anything in it, just a pillow and a blanket for sitting on the floor. I liked it that way. No noise, totally black, nothing human at all. I'd actually sit in that incredible black abyss, but it didn't feel bad. I was renewed in that place. It was scary to go there at first, because I had to take a leap of faith into something that was unknown. But when I learned to trust the abyss, it was amazing. I recognized it as home. It is my center, my core. I can trust the abyss because I'm never alone there.

I used to leave soothing music on to fill my home with healing vibrations while I was gone. Coming home to those vibrations helped me a lot.

Prayer helped me a lot, too. I learned that my prayers are answered more quickly when I pray in calmness, from my center. Grace comes to me more easily when I have surrendered.

Another turning point was when I felt ready to let go of my grief, and I realized I needed to become more involved in community in order to move forward in my life. I sold my house and moved here, to the Ananda Community, where I knew many people. After living alone for so long, I was just overwhelmed by having people around me all the time. It was too intense for a while, so I had to post notes on my door, saying that I was in seclusion for a week or two, to claim my time.

I've learned that setting boundaries is so important to my health. It's an important part of what keeps me centered and in touch with my personal power. Women are taught to be givers, to put their boundaries out too far. By doing that we betray ourselves and give away our personal power. We're afraid to say no, afraid to protect ourselves for fear that we will be rejected or abandoned. We wind up giving away too much of ourselves and feeling victimized. That throws us out of balance.

For me, setting boundaries means to love myself enough to stand up for what is right for me, and for what I need, even though sometimes I feel so alone when I am true to myself. That is when my heart is open and receptive to healing.

I believe that everyone has the ability to cultivate a receptive heart. And when we do, other people with open hearts are attracted to us.

John Pruitt
Seattle, Washington

Best Paint is a small Seattle company dedicated to producing safe paint products with a minimum of VOCs. Located in my neighborhood, this gem of a resource is owned and operated by co-founders John Pruitt and John Todd, two men who became chemically sensitive while working in the paint industry. Best Paint is advertised almost solely by word of mouth, and is carried only by a few retail outlets in Seattle; special orders are shipped to environmentally ill consumers nationwide. The two owners are always busy making paint or pouring energy into research and development of safe paint products.

I don't care who you are, if you expose yourself to toxic products over a period of time, it will get you. There's no getting around it.

I started painting about 1980. We did a lot of architectural finishes, finishes with cyanide in them, things like that. Sometimes we burned old paint to remove it. When you burn paint it changes the composition. Not even the manufacturer can tell you what the composition will be once you heat it. We used paint thinner to get oil-based paint off our skin. That just zaps into the bloodstream.

After I'd been painting for about seven years, I started reacting to some of the finishes I used. I started getting dizzy, things like that. I also found out I had liver damage. The doctor wanted to know if I was a heavy drinker. I wasn't a heavy drinker, but I had liver damage. I've learned that that is common among painters.

Just being around certain chemicals now, I can feel them burning my skin. Low levels, high levels—solvents in any amount really do a job on me. I can walk in a place and tell if there are solvents there. If there are, I just leave. I'm mostly sensitive to paint products. Anything with solvents. Fingernail polish remover, marking pens— those kinds of things almost knock me out. I can't be around them. I made one mark in a book with a highlighter, and that was it. Oh man, I got real dizzy. I put the cap back on and got rid of it.

I knew I had to do something different, that I wasn't going to paint anymore. I ran into John Todd. He and his brothers had a paint manufacturing business at that time. We talked about trying to make a paint that didn't make people sick. We got together and decided to try to make a product that was nontoxic. We started in 1989 and it took us about two years to come up with something. We're still working on it, adding and improving products.

There's a definite need. We get calls all the time from people who put up paint and—kaboom!—they've got problems. They can't go in their house. They don't know where to start to get help. If you're not getting a newsletter and don't belong to some supportive organization, it's really hard to just be out there on your own with this. I

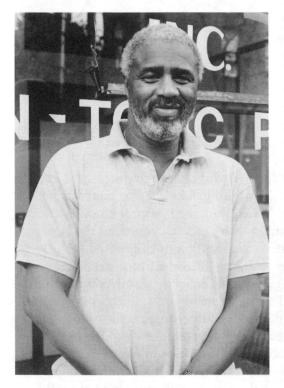

understand and I do what I can. I give them what little advice I have. I tell them everybody is different and you have to test everything and find out for yourself what will work for you. We don't try to sell them paint, we ask them to take a sample and try it first. I tell them, "You've got to find something that will work for you, and to keep your exposures down. Because the more exposures you have, the worse off you're going to be later on in life."

I've met people who were sealed into their homes, where they've got tape around their doors. They call us because something traumatic is going on and they need help. One lady was taped into her apartment. They were painting the outer walls and she was worried about what kind of paint they were going to use. This was her haven and she can't go outside. She called me for advice. A lot of times they want me to talk to the painter or to the people who own the building. Most are very receptive, some aren't. In the end they'll go along with me—at least on one portion of the job. They might think it's crazy, but they'll do it. They won't believe the resident. But I'm sort of a neutral party, so it works.

I think becoming chemically sensitive is a long process. Longer for some than for others. There are a lot of people who are chemically sensitive working right now in industry.

Matthew and Danielle Malcolm Camano Island, Washington

Matthew and Danielle Malcolm inherited allergies and a genetic predisposition for chemical sensitivities from their mother, and possibly their father. Their mother, Kathy, was sick with allergies, colds, tonsillitis and strep throat almost constantly as a child in Southern California. She also remembers feeling ill a lot in her parents' machine shop, where she spent a lot of time as a child. As an adult she pursued a career in photography and graphic arts, frequently using her bare hands to mix and use many chemicals. While working in that field Kathy had three miscarriages before her successful pregnancy with Matthew. When he was six weeks old the family moved into a new home with fresh paint and new carpeting throughout. Because the carpeting was flawed, a year later it was all replaced with more new carpeting.

As an infant Matthew developed rashes when he crawled on the carpeting, he cried inconsolably for no apparent reason, and rarely slept for more than forty-five minutes at a time. Kathy tried for several months to breast-feed him, but that did not provide enough nutrition for him. Looking back, she is horrified to realize that her breast milk contained high levels of toxic chemicals. Matthew's father was extremely allergic to milk as a child, an allergy which Matthew apparently inherited. When breast milk wasn't enough and he couldn't drink cow's milk without getting sick he was fed soy and goat's milk. When Matthew was nine months old an allergist in Arizona told Kathy he was allergic to "everything" and the family should move to a different climate. They relocated to a brand new, air-tight apartment in the Pacific Northwest, thinking it would be free of mold and dust and other traditional allergens. They were still oblivious to the effects of chemicals off-gassing from the new construction materials and carpeting. They stayed inside with the air conditioning on and the windows closed. Kathy developed bronchitis and coughed so hard she broke a rib. By then she had Danielle, who was on antihistamines at the age of three months. They all became sicker and sicker. Even-

tually Kathy learned from a doctor that they all had MCS in addition to traditional allergies.

Matthew was twelve years old and in the sixth grade at the time of this interview. His grades range from A+ to F, depending on his exposures to chemicals. When he is not having a chemical reaction his work is at the A and B level. If someone in the room is wearing a fragrance, or if he is reacting to some other exposure, he can barely pass a true-false examination, and his performance is even poorer on assignments requiring more complex thinking. On days when he is recovering from a previous exposure his condition is reflected by his work performance at a C level. Some teachers do not understand this correlation between chemical exposures and his school performance. He is in special education classes because he is considered "medically challenged" and he has a diagnosis of attention deficit disorder.

Matthew is especially reactive to soy products, dairy, chocolate, preservatives, fragrances, formaldehyde and diesel fumes. As a small boy he would develop a stuffy nose within minutes of eating dairy products, and by morning he would have a sinus infection. Other foods and chemicals—soy, chocolate and formaldehyde, for example—caused him to behave violently. His tolerance to those triggers has improved by taking antigens.

In the following narrative Matthew mentions an incident when he was teased about being allergic to chocolate. His mother explained to me that what had happened was that he had eaten chocolate in school, and in a reaction he had acted out so badly in class that the other students all were angry at him. His mother apologized to his classmates for his behavior and explained that it was caused by a reaction to the chocolate he had eaten. But instead of leading to forgiveness and compassion, his classmates used the information to hurt him.

In retrospect, Matthew's mother realizes that he was probably chemically sensitive at birth, but it was years before they understood the cause of his erratic, hyperactive, sometimes violent behavior. Because there seemed to be no rhyme or reason to his behaviors all that time, Matthew developed a poor self-image, impaired social skills, and a reputation for being difficult.

Although I found it difficult to keep Matthew focused during our interview, I also found that beneath his somewhat chaotic exterior is a deep, sweet boy with commitment and perseverance. With the hope that he could overcome his intolerance to certain foods, for years he followed a strict diet when most kids would have given in to temptations. He still willingly follows a strict diet and restricted lifestyle because he doesn't like how he feels during a reaction. But he's angry that he doesn't seem to receive much of a reward for his efforts.

In order to cope with the emotional pain and rejection he has suffered, his imagination has flourished. He is a creative writer and hopes to one day be a published author.

Danielle, nine years old when interviewed, enjoys playing the piano and recorder, and making colorful origami animals. Ordinarily even-tempered, Danielle experiences dramatic physical and emotional reactions from exposure to perfumes and other chemicals, and from eating certain foods containing additives and allergens. Her reactions include nosebleeds, muscle aches, headaches, crying spells and irritability.

Matthew

When I'm going to sleep at night I think about going to a movie or eating a hamburger with friends. No normal kids thinks about these things because they just happen to them. I dream of those things.

My mom told me that my allergies would all be gone by the time I was eight years old. When I was finally eight and she said I still couldn't have this or that, I said, "Noooooo!" I get angry with the guy [God] up there.

I also get angry when kids tease me at school. Like, when people ask me, "Are you allergic to water?" I say, "I'm not allergic to water."

Last year was the worst for me. I picked on the girls that year because for my entire life they'd said, "You stupid person." Stuff like that. I usually ignored them, but then I got real angry.

Once my mom told everybody in my class that I was allergic to chocolate, and *baaad* things happened. They were so mean. They'd put chocolate right in my face. That I cannot take. I can resist candy—I ate chocolate just once in school. But I can't take the teasing sometimes. I got angry with them and lost my temper. And I was angry with my mom for a week.

I've been learning to control my temper. I practice with my mom.

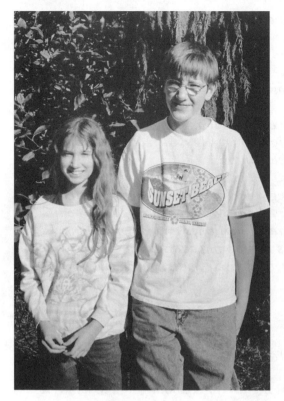

I can control my temper with her. The computer helps me with my anger too. With the computer you can let out your anger on all the guys that are "technically" picking on you. You can blow them to bits because they're not real people.

Now I'm in a new school and I have friends who don't make a big deal out of it when I take my pills. They made a big deal of it the first couple of days. I said I was taking vitamins. They said, "Oh, antibiotics." I said, "They're not antibiotics, they're vitamins." And that was the end of it.

My buddy is Eric. When the teacher gives out candy as a reward, I give mine to Eric. I call him a walking encyclopedia because he knows almost everything. One day the teacher said she had corrected our papers, and there were only two that were perfect. I pointed to Eric, and the teacher said one of them was Eric's. I was thinking the other one was going to be Melinda's. But the teacher said, "Matt." I got an A+, an even better grade than Eric got!

People with MCS have big temptations. I'm the good guy who doesn't eat the bad stuff. It's the guilt, the little thing that eats inside you, that I don't like. I was recently offered a cookie and ice cream, and I said no.

I don't like how I feel if I eat things I'm not supposed to. Every year I've gotten a horrible disease. Last year I had a 104-degree temperature and I was home for a month. I wasn't scared. The scary part was going back to school because I had piles and piles and piles of work.

My sister eats things she's not supposed to, and we can tell by her reactions.

I say, be the good guy. It makes you feel better inside and gives you something to tease your brother or sister about if they give in to temptation.

Danielle

When I smell perfume I get sick. I get headaches and sometimes my nose bleeds. One time when we were in reading groups at school, I opened a brand new book and it smelled so strong, I thought I was going to pass out. My friends Ashley and Libby were in my group. I said, "Can you guys read for me? I can't stand the book." They said okay.

I can't go to places where my friends go, like the movies or the mall; I've gone to a mall four or six times in my life. I can't go over to other kids' houses, I can't eat chocolate, and I can't buy school lunches.

If one of my friends wears something that smells and it bothers me, they go into the bathroom and rinse it off. That helps a little bit because then it's not so strong. And sometimes they just try to stay a distance away from me, but we can still play.

The first day at my new school I didn't tell anybody. I decided to tell them on the second day of school, when I knew they weren't going to ditch me. I kind of told one of my friends a little bit at a time—like, I'm allergic to this and I'm allergic that—so she didn't freak all at once.

It's not very easy having this problem, because kids at school tease me. I don't want to get pushed around so I just say, "You wouldn't have such a big mouth if I punched you!" That backs them off. People will stop bugging you if you stand up for yourself. Sometimes I stand up for my friends, too.

Terri Crawford Hansen
Whidbey Island, Washington

Terri Crawford Hansen is a bright and warm individual whose life has changed dramatically—in both positive and negative direc-

tions—as a result of chronic fatigue and MCS. Her marriage ended in divorce. She lost custody of her daughter. She developed a mental illness. And she found her identity.

Terri was a stranger to her Indian heritage in her youth. While visiting a pueblo for the first time as a young adult, she felt a kinship with the Indians, which she could not express. Today her Indian roots shape her life and soul, providing her with healing rituals that help her to cope with her illness. She is an internationally known investigative reporter of chemical injury in the Native American community.

Terri courageously disclosed that she suffers from bipolar disorder, a mental illness which her physician attributes to MCS. It was not the first time I had heard of this theory. Terri had no history of mental illness prior to the onset of her chronic fatigue and MCS.

As a child growing up in Portland, Oregon, she sometimes suffered from eczema and was prone to react to poison oak. Other than that, she was a healthy child, the oldest of five. Terri has a daughter who is seven years old. Without a trace of anger, fear or bitterness in her voice, she told me her story over a cup of tea in the CyberCafe bookstore on Whidbey Island.

I'm a newspaperwoman and I always have been. I went to work for the *Oregonian* when I was twenty. I was outgoing and very effective. I could do anything handed to me. I worked in advertising, composing, the newsroom and on the copy desk. After I got sick I wasn't able to do anything, because my brain wouldn't function.

I started getting sick during a third remodeling at work. It involved the installation of a lot of partitions that were off-gassing formaldehyde. I was engulfed in it. The nerves swelled up in my joints in my elbows, knees, wrists and heels. It's called peripheral polyneuropathy or nerve entrapments. It's like carpal tunnel syndrome. I didn't associate my illness with the remodeling, at the time. I thought it was from ergonomics. I took numerous leaves and would start to improve, then I'd get sick again when I went back to work. In '92 I quit work entirely and went on disability.

I feel fortunate that I was born an Indian, because I have something tangible that nourishes my spirit. I follow the Indian way. I can have a vision, and when I tell another Indian person about my vision it is not questioned. I can talk to the spirits. I can ask questions, and then I am at peace because I know my answers will be there. They may not come in the next day or two, but they will come. And whatever is supposed to happen for me will.

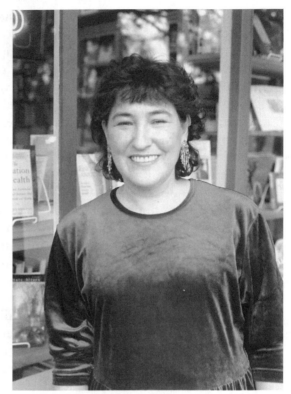

I have rituals. I pray daily. And every morning and every evening I burn and smudge sage or sweetgrass to purify myself and my home. Sage and sweetgrass are sacred to Indians. Sometimes I gather and bundle my own. Cedar is more sacred in the Northwest, but I can't work with it because it makes me sick.

I go to sweats. At first the sweat makes me feel worse, because I'm detoxing chemicals. Then I feel better. The closest one I know of is at the Suquamish Reservation. That's a ferry ride across to Port Townsend, and then a drive down to the reservation. I could travel a lot more if I wasn't sick.

Prior to getting sick I had three miscarriages, all during the first trimester. After the second one the doctors started running tests, and nothing was found. Before that, I'd never seen the inside of a hospital. Eventually I gave birth. My baby weighed only five pounds, fifteen ounces. By then I had been diagnosed with chronic fatigue syndrome. I took twelve weeks off from work when my baby was born. She was born with a rash all over her body, and she immediately developed colic—which was hard to live with. Looking back, I can see that symptoms she experienced as an infant were symptoms of MCS. In preschool her hands and feet turned purple. She had developed Raynaud's disease, which I have, too. But now she is okay; I think she's in remission. She doesn't have any food allergies or MCS, and I hope she doesn't get it.

After I had to quit working, my daughter and I would go to the beach for a few days at a time. I loved the beach and felt better there. Eventually my husband and I decided to live near the beach. He was an attorney, and after we moved he set up his practice in a brand new office. Every time I visited him at that office I became violently ill. That's how I finally figured out that I was chemically sensitive. I'd get migraine headaches and dizzy spells, and sometimes I would vomit. I'd get so sick that I couldn't even talk. The dizzy spells were horrendous. I've had them off and on since then, after chemical exposures. Once I was so dizzy that I fell trying to get up from my bed. That's when I quit using detergents, household cleaners, hair spray and deodorant.

Fragrances don't seem to bother me as much as other chemicals. Formaldehyde is the worst for me. I have to stay away from new carpeting and new or remodeled buildings. Car exhaust is another one. And chlorine. Once when I went to the doctor they put me in a robe that had been washed with bleach, and I got sick right there in the doctor's office from wearing it.

I've been diagnosed with bipolar disorder. I just went through a depression, but now I'm feeling better. The problem with bipolar is that when you are treated for depression it can set off a manic episode. I have to be really careful. I've been hospitalized four times with manic episodes. I was told by a doctor that my bipolar disorder is an imbalance in brain chemistry caused by chemical exposures.

I've had Indian people tell me to quit using the white man's medicine and use only traditional herbs. I try to explain that I'm not able to. If I stopped taking my medication I'd probably become manic again. And, I've been told that if I go off the medication there's a good chance that it wouldn't work for me again if went back to it. I'm grateful that I can tolerate normal doses of medications, unlike some people with MCS. But I like to take as few as possible. I do take medication for the nerve entrapments because, even though I look okay, it would be very difficult for me to walk very far and to get around if I didn't take that medication.

On three different occasions my hair has fallen out in clumps. It used to be long, down to my waist. I'd be sitting there writing and you could see my hair blanketing the carpet behind me. I saw a dermatologist, who couldn't find anything wrong with me. Eventually I had to cut my hair short because it was so thin and strange-looking. I hated to cut it because long hair is a part of my culture. You can tell by looking at another Indian whether or not they are traditional by the length of their hair. If they wear their hair in a traditional manner, then you know they are of a like mind and you feel a kinship with them. Cutting my hair has affected my relationships with other Indian women. Now I feel I have to go the extra mile to reassure them that I am a traditional Indian woman.

My illness has affected my relationships in many ways. It affected my marriage, which ended in divorce. I can't say that I blame my husband for leaving. It was a very difficult situation. He took my daughter to live with him because I am too ill to care for her on a full-time basis. I see her on Tuesdays, Fridays and Saturdays. We have a co-parenting plan that would allow me to see her more often, but I can't. She's seven, and she requires a lot of care. If I'm having a bad day, it's very difficult. I miss having a family. That's real sad and hard for me to talk about.

In many ways my life has changed for the better. It wasn't until after I quit my job that I became Indian. After I had to quit my job, I started volunteering in the Indian community. That was good for me, to go back to my roots. My mother was all Indian. She was removed from the reservation at the age of three because her mother died. She was adopted by a family in Portland and never developed an interest in her Indian heritage. I'm the oldest of five children. When I was eighteen I went back to enroll us at the Winnebago of Nebraska reservation.

While volunteering in the Indian community I noticed that a large part of the population was sick, and no one knew what was causing it. When they started talking to me about their symptoms, I recognized it as MCS. I've gotten quite a few of them to a doctor. It was like my own private war.

Since then doctors and researchers have found evidence that the prevalence of MCS is higher in the Indian community than in the general population. A local doctor on the Seattle Indian Board began volunteering in the Indian community when he went into semi-retirement, and he noticed that the Indian people were getting sick at a much higher rate than the general population. He determined they were sick from multiple chemical sensitivity. Another doctor told me about a survey done by the Department of Health in New Mexico, showing that 31 percent of the Native Americans surveyed identified themselves as chemically sensitive, compared to 17 percent in the general population. I was told that number is conservative because they were unable to reach a lot of the poorer, isolated Indians.

Native Americans may be more susceptible to MCS because of a P450 enzyme deficiency; this enzyme is needed to break down toxic chemicals in the body. Another factor that contributes to poor health in Indian communities is that more toxic wastes are dumped on reservations than anywhere else in the United States.

When I got involved in the Indian community I started publishing a tabloid called *The Portland Indian News*. One story I published was called "Does MCS Affect American Indians in Higher Numbers?" The story ended with a big question mark, and was picked up by *News from Indian Country*, a bimonthly Native paper circulated in all fifty states, the Canadian provinces and eight foreign countries.

News from Indian Country also published a story I wrote about the health problems of the Shoalwater Bay tribe and the basket weavers of California. The Shoalwater Indians live on a small reservation in Washington, with chemical poisoning on all sides, and is suffering from an unusually large number of miscarriages, still births, and cases of chronic fatigue syndrome. The basket weavers formed an organization eleven years ago because they were getting sick from the native grasses they harvested in the forests and along the roadsides, areas that had been sprayed with pesticides; they were getting sick from flattening the grasses between their teeth. I also told stories about groups of Indians living along the Columbia, one of the filthiest rivers in the country from the release of so much dioxins. Growing up in Portland, I spent a lot of time playing in the Columbia River.

Writing helps me to cope with living with MCS, with the loneliness and isolation that I feel. At one time I was the Pacific Northwest bureau chief for *News from Indian County*, but I had to cut back because of my health. I'm still writing for them.

If I'm having a bad day I sometimes still write, unless a reaction to a chemical is affecting my brain. When I can't think clearly, I can't write. And sometimes I feel so apathetic that I can't write. But I'm thankful that I have the skill. I think education is so important to prevent others from getting this illness. I believe that chronic fatigue syndrome, fibromyalgia, sick building syndrome and similar conditions with other names are all forms of MCS. They'll find that out with more studies. People just don't know what's wrong with them. They think they've got asthma, depression, attention deficit disorder and a lot of other problems that can be related to chemical exposures.

I've met a lot of neat people who have this illness and who are survivors, people who care about other people, people who have become activists. I've seen more reconciliation than anger. People with MCS don't want to just sit there, they want to help. A lot of people are putting out newsletters, writing books and disseminating information. I started a nonprofit organization called The National American Indian Environmental Illness Foundation. I mail my brochure and free materials by request.

I wish I never would have gotten MCS. But it happened. And I went back to my roots.

Canadian Stories

We tell and retell our stories, since they have levels of meaning which cannot be completely captured in a single telling.—From *Winter Grace* by Kathleen Fischer

Karen Forbes
Victoria, British Columbia

When I first contacted Karen Forbes I was struck by her positive attitude. She suggested I also talk to Jean MacKenzie and Katy Young—whose stories are included in this volume—and told me they all were aiming for complete recovery from MCS. At that point I had never heard of anyone who was completely recovered from MCS, and I wasn't sure that it was possible. By the time I left Victoria I was convinced that anything is possible when the synergy of three dynamic women is in action.

Karen, Jean and Katy enjoy a remarkable camaraderie and have been successful in their efforts to develop resources for people with MCS on Vancouver Island. They had almost nothing in common prior to MCS, and much of their advocacy work is done individually. Just knowing the other two are nearby and persevering helps to energize them.

Karen grew up on a prairie in Regina, Saskatchewan, where pesticides were sprayed regularly. To her knowledge, the only allergy she had as a child was to milk. At age sixteen she moved to Victoria with her family, to the home where she resides today.

When I interviewed Karen she was editor of the Ecological Health Alliance newsletter and a leader of the Victoria area MCS support group. She is petite and soft-spoken but not quiet.

An element of surprise I enjoyed on this trip was a chemical-free bed and breakfast found serendipitously on a country road not far from Karen's home.

It's like an avalanche effect. You get all these assaults and you get sick, but you don't believe this is happening. Then there's one stone too many and the whole thing tumbles down and, unless you stop it, you hit bottom.

My background is in hairdressing, you see, so I was working in a chemical industry. When I look back through pictures that I have, I can see the dark circles under my eyes and the puffy weight. So, I realize now that I was probably allergic to a lot of different things then, but I didn't know it.

Ten or fifteen years into hairdressing, I started working for the research and development department of a large cosmetic company in addition to working in a salon. They sent me to salons to teach about the chemistry of hair products. I was very interested in the chemistry end of it. That's not something normally taught to a hairdresser. Most hairdressers don't know what they're using or what they're exposed to. That's starting to change, now. But when I first started, I had no idea what was in these products.

Working for this company, I had an opportunity to go to an educational seminar in Florida. While I was there I woke up with what I thought was the worst cold I'd ever had. My head was splitting, I could hardly lift it off the pillow. My chest was heavy. I got the chills. I was so sick. I took some aspirin and had some breakfast and tried to pull myself together. I had just finished the seminar and was traveling to the other coast. When I got there and checked into a motel I told them I was sick and didn't know how long I'd be there, that it was probably going to take me a day or two to kick this. After taking one look at me they were so worried that they sent someone to check on me every three hours. I stood in the shower until I'd drained the hot water tank and had the heat up as high as it could go. I couldn't get warm. I was the sickest I'd ever been. I knew I had to eat, so the next day I went to a restaurant right next door. I was so out of it that I didn't realize it was such a ritzy place. I was wearing jeans that looked like I'd slept in them—which I had! But they were really kind and sat me at a nice table. After I ate some fish I felt a little better. But when I came back to Canada I still didn't completely recover. I had chronic fatigue. I went to doctors and everybody kept telling me I had the flu. This went on for months and months. I finally went to a doctor who said that parasites were a part of the problem.

The cure was worse than the parasites. I took a medication that wiped out my immune system. I turned gray. I couldn't work. I couldn't eat. This happened two weeks before I was supposed to go to New Zealand. And I still went. But, oh, God, I was sick.

In New Zealand I met a homeopathist who helped me. That's how I was able to travel and to get back to Canada. When I came back I tried to work and couldn't. I spent another eight months off work, thinking I was still trying to get over an antibiotic reaction. Then I went back to work again, back to working with chemicals. At that time my employer was renovating the salon. They did everything you can think of—new carpeting, new paint, you name it. I had no idea those things were affecting me. I didn't do too badly during the renovations. My body resisted and resisted, then just started to break down. One day my assistant sprayed Windex on my mirror and I couldn't breathe. So that was it, no more Windex. Windex went.

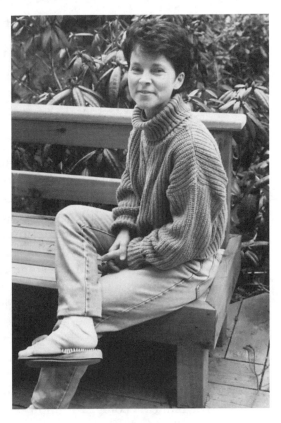

Then it was food. When I ate certain foods I'd get a racing, irregular heartbeat and everything would speed up. I'd get hot and flushed, and it was hard to breathe. When it was over I'd get diarrhea, my feet would be cold, and I would be totally drained. That's enough to make you not want to eat. You sure can't take too many of those episodes before you can't cope with everyday life.

The food sensitivities started moving closer together. I began to lose my tolerance to more foods every day, and it just started to snowball.

I still didn't know the chemicals bothered me. The doctor kept telling me I had the flu. But I didn't have the flu. I went to see another doctor who understood environmental illness and MCS. She said, "You have to quit your job now. Not tomorrow. Now."

So I quit my job, and I realized chemicals had something to do with what was going on, but I didn't know to what extent. Nor did

I know how much sicker I would get trying to recover. That wasn't the end of it at all.

My doctor wanted me to see the admitting physician at the mental institution to rule out an eating disorder. I had worked in a facility for kids that are mentally disturbed, so I knew what the admitting sequence was–that they'd try to push as many buttons as possible. I knew that if I was having a chemical reaction when I was interviewed I wouldn't be able to think clearly, and I might appear overly emotional. The risk was that they would assume my reactions were caused by a mental illness. I also knew that if I played the game right I could get what I wanted—a requisition to see the clinical ecologist in Vancouver for allergy testing. Fortunately, on the day of my appointment I was not in a reaction and I was feeling stable. I told the interviewer that I wanted a referral to a clinical ecologist for food allergy testing, and that if for some reason the testing did not turn up anything I was willing to entertain the idea that I had an eating disorder or that I was crazy. I also asked for a backup requisition for the food disorder program, to have me committed if the clinical ecologist did not believe that my illness was caused by food allergies. That's scary! But I had a gut feeling I had food allergies, and I knew a traditional allergist would turn up nothing. I think I was down to eating potatoes and cauliflower at that time.

The clinical ecologist found that I had many food and chemical sensitivities. My lowest point came after I started a desensitization treatment program, because that is when I became the most hypersensitive. Science fiction is what it was like. Things got really bizarre. I couldn't have contact with people. I had to be sort of quarantined. At one point I couldn't go into the grocery store because all I'd smell was the cleaners. My partner, Mark, couldn't even cook for a long time because of the reactions I'd get from the food smells. So there were a lot of inconveniences.

I was afraid my relationship with Mark might not survive the worst periods of my MCS. I was afraid he wouldn't understand that depression and anger are chemical reactions.

I try to be aware of what's happening and how I feel, and I verbalize it. When I'm reacting to chemicals and I feel angry, I try to figure out if there's really something to be angry about or if it's part of my chemical reaction. I tell Mark to give me a wide berth when I'm feeling bad. That's the only way we've survived this. Communication is definitely the key.

Three or four months into my desensitization we had a pesticide spill in our water supply. We didn't know about it until one day when I was having trouble tolerating water. I spent all day cooking food and throwing it out. I was worried. I was down to sixty-five pounds. I had to eat. I couldn't even eat rice cooked in water. And there was very little organic produce available here at that time, which is the only produce I could tolerate.

For a two-year period I was incoherent a lot of the time. Most of that time I don't even remember, my brain was so scrambled. Even when I thought I was speaking normally, I wasn't. That's scary!

My family was supportive. We came from an area where there are a lot of toxic chemicals and people get pesticide poisoning. We also lived in an area where you had somebody come in and dowse if you had water problems. Dowsing was a normal thing, not crazy.

When my parents come here they have to detox their clothes because they're used to using fabric softener. They also have to use the shampoo and personal care products I provide because I get sick from their shampoo and other things they are accustomed to using.

Mark's family has had more trouble accepting my illness. His mother and sister both are nurses who received conventional training. To them, clinical ecologists and little vials of homeopathic remedies seem crazy.

Most people don't understand at all what happens to you with this illness. Your social life is virtually nil, really. You can lose your livelihood, which is a big loss for most people because what we do for a living is often our identity. For me, my job was also a social network. At the time when I had to quit working I didn't feel that it was all that important, because I was coping with survival. I didn't worry about it. But when I started to get well I realized how much I had lost. Being seriously ill for a long time, I've had to operate in a fight or flight condition. It's tough to get out of that when your health begins to improve. In our support group I see people who have fought for so long that they can't get out of that cycle even if they've gotten considerably better. They're fighting for housing, fighting for this or that. To stay in that mode, you get sicker because when you're in that mode the body manufactures chemicals which are not good for you.

When I started to get better I realized I was chronically depressed. I felt numb. I knew that if I let it go further than that, I wouldn't want to get out of bed. I knew that wasn't a good place to be, that

I was still in the flight or fight cycle. I always had a strong sense of self, and I wanted to get well. So I knew to seek counseling. I spent three years with a very good counselor who helped me through some of that stress. Now depression isn't a big problem for me.

My counselor's specialty was eating disorders, which is one of the reasons I wanted to see her. Even though I knew my illness wasn't caused by an eating disorder, food was still part of the problem. There were some foods that I was not reacting to at that point, but I didn't know how to go back to eating them. Heavens—when you have a cardiovascular attack, you bet you're afraid to eat again! But this counselor helped me through that fear. Something else that has helped me is kinesiology. I have used that to learn how to heal my body from the trauma I've experienced with this illness.

Constant change is another challenge of living with MCS. I can figure out what works for me right now, but that doesn't mean that's going to work a month from now. It'll change again according to my health and my tolerance. I had a real hard time with that for a long time.

Right now I'm especially reactive to cleaners and dish soaps. I had a dish soap that I tolerated for a few months, and now I've lost that. I'm still reactive to normal water, so I can't eat in restaurants because the food is cooked in water—and most restaurants have gas stoves, and I'm not very tolerant of gas. I have a stainless steel distiller I transport around with me. We have a little trailer, and I have to travel with my distiller and a two-burner electric stove. The trailer has a gas stove, which we don't use, and it has a rubberized liner which caused problems for me so we've sealed it the best we can. We can't park in the sun because heat bakes the rubber and causes it to off-gas fumes that make me sick.

In my opinion, the ability to accept change is critical to living with MCS. If you aren't willing to try something different, you can paint yourself into a corner with very few options. That's a scary place to be.

I have found that it helps me to stay calm and let my body and adrenals rest. That alone can make a difference. The more often I can do that, the better. And for me, a lot of getting well is learning how to set boundaries. If I don't take care of myself, I'm not going to get better. I've had to learn when I've had enough, when to say no, when I'm too tired to do any more regardless of what else is on my list.

Spirituality and creativity are also important parts of my recovery program. I can't focus just on housing and food issues. There has to be more. So I've started working with papier-mâché and rubber stamps and embossing, even though I have to wear a mask when I use some of the materials. Exercise is important, too. I have a little rebounder that I like. The rebounder is a good way to get my system moving if I can't get outside. When I can, I garden and mow the lawn—with an electric lawnmower.

After I got so sick my worst fear, for years, was being a bag lady. That's a pretty valid fear for many of us who have been ill for a long time. I've talked to many people who don't have anyone to look after them, and can't find a safe place to live. We're making progress on that front in Victoria, but it's slow. B.C. Housing has designated housing for people with MCS. So far two apartments have been made available. But those who need them most can't move in because the apartments are new and haven't off-gassed, and one of them is downwind from the laundry unit.

It's hard to give people hope. We tell people who are looking for safe housing to look at apartment buildings that have hardwood floors and to contact churches that provide public housing. But a lot of these buildings are sprayed with pesticides, so you have to find out if they only spray the storage areas or all the floors. Some of our people have gone into rooms rented in private homes. There the problem is that you have communal laundries and bathrooms which you might have to decontaminate each time you use them. It's not easy. One of the only ways you can get around it is to try to get well so you can tolerate more. The better I've gotten, the more I can tolerate and the more options there are open to me.

It was almost four years after I became ill that I was able to go out without becoming totally incapacitated. I went to a bridal shower where nobody wore perfume. They knew I couldn't be there otherwise. That was a big thing for me. Now I can go to movies—not many people in our group can handle that one. I pay for it, somewhat, but I can manage it. The price I pay depends on how strong I am on the day that I go. There are a lot of places I go, but when I come home I have to take off my clothes, put them in the laundry and take a shower to get rid of all the scents I've picked up. I pretty much do what I want now, but I realize there are limits to how long I can do it without getting sick. My life is still far from what most people consider normal.

Mark teaches hang gliding. And when he teaches people how to land he tells them not to look at trees, because where you look is exactly where you're going to land. I feel that I'm looking in the right direction as a person with MCS. I'm still in transition, but I've got a life.

Jean MacKenzie
Victoria, British Columbia

When I first began this book I had never heard of anyone who had recovered from MCS. Then I met Jean MacKenzie. More than fifteen years ago she was severely disabled by MCS, and was in isolation for several years. Today she enjoys a full life with very few restrictions, devoting a great deal of time and energy to supporting others suffering from the illness, and to MCS education and activism.

Jean is a co-founder of Ecological Health Alliance, a group providing education and support to people with MCS in Victoria. Two years ago the group joined with a national organization and is now the British Columbia branch of the Allergy and Environmental Health Association of Canada. A native of Vancouver, Jean has lived on Vancouver Island with her husband for more than forty years.

I used to be quite shy and retiring, but now I'm quite feisty. Well, there's something to be feisty about. Now I don't care what other people think. I've gotten past that.

Early on, at about age fourteen, I had skin reactions to things like elastic and that sort of thing. I had worked a summer job as a silk presser in a dry cleaning establishment, and things began to bother me increasingly. Later I was doing window dressings and signs, and that involved a lot of solvents. I didn't realize what I was doing to myself. And I began to have a lot of trouble. Of course I never knew what it was.

I had lower back pain for years. Everybody said it was arthritis and gave me pills to take. I was taking very high doses of medications and barely holding my own. Then my stomach began to act up, of course, because of the medications. So I had to get out of that.

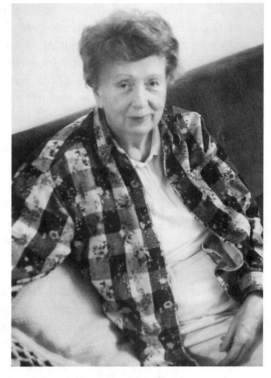

I went to the library and found a book about alternative ways of dealing with arthritis. It talked about muscle testing to identify foods and other substances that might be causing adverse reactions, and the nightshades—the food family that includes potatoes, tomatoes and peppers—those sorts of things. It really sounded weird. I'd never heard of anything like that. But I thought, what the heck! So I had some muscle testing and—whamo!–down went my arm. I thought, okay, I can give up potatoes for a while; let's just see what happens. And within a week I had cut the medication by half, and in a month I was off it completely. It was just remarkable.

Then I realized there was more going on. I went to work in my husband's office, which, unfortunately, was over a kitchen cabinet shop. They used a lot of solvents, and the fumes came into our office. I began to get really sick, and I phoned up an allergist for an appointment. I was told they wouldn't give me an appointment because it sounded like I was chemically sensitive and there was no cure for that. So I said to myself, I'll find a cure!

I was mad as hell, but quite determined that I was going to get out of it. I really felt that I could get better. I did a lot of reading. Theron Randolph's book, *An Alternative Approach to Allergies*, was very helpful, of course, in the beginning stages.

When I realized that I was even reacting to the drapes in my house, I told my husband we had to strip the house of everything.

I said, "This is what we have to do whether you like it or not." Most of the furniture went into storage and we put up cotton sheets in place of the drapes. I bought all cotton clothes. I was wearing nothing but white cotton, and I looked like a spook! I had a mattress made with no rubber in it at all. I was reacting to a lot of foods, so I used to drive around trying to find something I could eat.

At first my husband didn't believe I was reacting to all these things. But he went along with me and finally saw that the changes we made were having a positive effect on my health. He's been tremendous. I couldn't have done it without him sticking with me. Lots of husbands go the other way.

If I hadn't had that kind of support, I don't think I would have recovered. I couldn't work, so I wouldn't have had the money for all the treatments that have helped me. We decided at the beginning that we wouldn't add up how much it cost us. I was going to get better no matter what. I don't even like to think about how much it's cost. Thousands and thousands of dollars for treatments, supplements and all the various things that we've tried.

We went into isolation for several years. It was very hard on my husband. I feel like it has affected his life. He was going out and about, but he didn't really want to go if I couldn't go because he is a conscionable soul. It kept us from traveling and doing a lot of things we wanted to do. We missed a lot, but we've gained a lot of things, too. And we've learned a lot. Oh, man, we've learned a lot. Not all things that we wanted to learn, but that's all right, that's what life's all about.

Other people were sympathetic but they didn't understand it at all. There was always the feeling that Jean had gotten "a little funny," you know. I knew that people didn't understand and I didn't blame them. I probably internalized a lot of feelings that other people might give vent to. Whether that's bad or good, I'm not sure. I relied mostly on myself. I knew it wasn't in my head, I knew it in my bones.

I did a lot of inner work, a lot of spiritual work that I probably wouldn't have if I'd just been sailing blithely through life. Because when you get hit with this you look where your foundations are, because you need the foundations. That has certainly been true for me.

When I was in the depths of despair I went for prayer and the laying on of hands with friends. I did that quite frequently. That was what helped me to keep going. People do get healed in the most remarkable ways through Christian healing. For people who are not into religion there are other forms of energy healing, such as Reiki.

My belief is that energy is the blueprint of your body. In the Bible God says, "Before you were formed in the womb, I knew you." That means you were God's thought, you were energy before you were physical. To me that means that if there's an illness, there's something awry with your body energy. And if you can change that energy, then you can change the illness. That's where I'm coming from right now. So whether we are talking about Christianity or Reiki or Touch for Health, we are talking about alteration of body energy.

I believe those of us with MCS are sensitive because of our particular energy patterns. What makes you sick might be an energy pattern you inherited. I think that energy patterns can come down through the generations. Most of us who have chemical sensitivities probably have family members—or ancestors—who are or were affected to one degree or another, whether they admit that or not. My father was once stung by a bee and nearly died. My brother is very sensitive to cold. After swimming in a cold river he came out of the water with great welts all over himself, stopped breathing and nearly died.

In previous generations you just avoided whatever it was you were sensitive to. Now we are bombarded with chemicals we can't avoid, and they are affecting our energy patterns.

When I was going through the worst period of my illness I didn't know anyone else with MCS until my doctor called one day to ask if I would let a woman come to our house to take a bath. The doctor knew my house was nontoxic. That's when we got involved with another gal who was desperately ill with MCS. I said sure, if someone was in trouble to send them along. And this gal came along. She was in terrible shape, absolutely wiped. Her mother was her support person. They were living in their car. We ended up doing their laundry at our house for five years because they could not find a safe place to do laundry. We tried to take this gal to Vancouver for treatment. We had her on a ferry and had done our level best to keep her from being exposed to anything. We had her outside on the deck when a guy came by wearing aftershave, and she collapsed completely. It was horrifying. The whole trip was shot.

It turned out that this gal and other people were being affected by a great plume of black smoke that went up all over Victoria when the Department of National Defence was training firefighters. They were using diesel to start fires, and to extinguish the fires they used AFF foam [Aqueous Film Forming Foam]. We discovered that the foam is highly toxic, and in combustion with diesel it's lethal. So we began to lobby to get them to stop. It's been a major battle, but now they are using less toxic products.

More and more chemically sensitive people contacted us when they became aware of our efforts, so we decided to form a group. We persuaded the Capital Regional District health officer to back us up in a survey to establish there was a population of people here with environmental illness. We thought there might be twenty-five or so people. But we heard from people way up-island and in the interior and Vancouver. We stopped at two hundred and fifty. Many wrote on their survey forms, "You mean I'm not the only one?"

It's so important for people to hook up with somebody else who can tell them they're not crazy and who can give support and share information about treatments they've tried. MCS is a real fear-producing illness, so we need all the support we can get. I know fear. I've had it. But I've been able to drag myself out of it. I was afraid I wasn't going to be able to get well, despite my determination. When I lost my tolerance to so many foods, and my clothes, and my house and my friends, I began to wonder what was going to be left. It's real important that people connect to a support group of some kind. It's just too big for one person by themselves. Even if you've only got a little group of four or five people, it makes a big difference.

So many people with MCS feel absolutely devastated and alone because they don't know anybody else with the illness or because they are dealing with a doctor who doesn't know anything about it. They think the doctor is supposed to know. So when the doctor doesn't know and runs a bunch of tests and says nothing is wrong, says you're crazy, what do you do? It's really important to hook up with people who can give you support and information.

One of the biggest problems for people with MCS is housing. I hear from a lot of people who are having trouble living in apartments. People living in apartments are sitting ducks for all the neighbors' contaminants plus the cleaning materials used in the building. When you tell people it makes you sick, some get very defensive and nasty. Some will go out of their way to spray you with a fragrance or chemical just to see if you'll turn blue. We've had people being sent to the hospital in desperate conditions. All we can do is try to hold them up and speak on their behalf.

B.C. Housing is now working with our group to provide safe housing. We're just beginning that. I think we've just placed a second person. She's so terribly ill that she's terrified to move from where she is to another place.

A lot of people call our organization and ask, "Where can I go? Where can I live?" We can't recommend a place to go and be safe because everybody is different. There's very little we can offer but emotional support.

I think it's important to be flexible in looking for ways to wellness. And I think it's important to be judicious, as well. I don't advocate rushing from one doctor to another, from one treatment to another. But my theory is that everybody's got a piece of the elephant. When I'm bogged down and not getting anywhere trying to improve my health, it's time to start looking at another path. When I'm considering a treatment I compare notes with different people on my health team. I say, "What do you think about this? What do you think about that?" If I'm considering a new medication I test it very carefully before I take it, to make sure I'm not going to have a severe reaction to it.

It's important for me to keep a journal to record how I feel, the treatments I've tried and the results. Because when I'm having a reaction it seems like I've felt that way forever and I'm never going to get out of it. If I look back at my journal and realize it's only been two days that I've been in this mess, this gives me a bit more of a foundation. I can say to myself: It's only been two days and you didn't die yet, and I think you really did feel a little better today than you felt yesterday, so you're probably going to live through this one, Jean! I found that to be very helpful, because it's easy to drop into the fear cycle. And once I do that, my body starts putting out the wrong chemicals. It's very important to keep a hopeful attitude. Negative thoughts, as far as I can determine, generate adverse chemical results in my body.

It took me four or five years to get strong. Now I can go almost anywhere I want to, but I will not go into a carpet store. And if I see somebody coming along the street made up to the gills, I know they're loaded with fragrances and I avoid them. I also don't enjoy having people come to my home wearing fragrances. It wouldn't wipe me out. But I don't want to be exposed to toxic chemicals and I don't enjoy having the house smell or having to wash out my clothes after they depart.

Do I consider myself healed? Not completely. I've got a lot of work to do—a lot of interior work—because I believe that the way I think affects my health. My body believes every word I say and every thought I think.

There are so many desperate people out there with MCS. I tell them my story and all the things I can do now. I tell them I think they can get better. It may take a long time—barring any miracle, which we're all available for—but you can get better.

_____

Katy Young
Victoria, British Columbia

Katy Young is president of the Ecological Health Alliance, a branch of the Allergy and Environmental Health Association of Canada, providing information, education, resources and support to those with food and environmental sensitivities. She is a single mother of two young boys, both who are also chemically sensitive. Katy is an MCS activist and herbalist. She grows organic herbs, conducts garden tours and provides indoor air quality consultations in Victoria. As a child she lived in Edmonton and Vancouver, and moved to Vancouver Island at the age of twelve.

In this interview Katy shares her view that chemical exposures can lead to an inability to tolerate stress, to loss of mental functioning, to fear and to violence. Since I met with her, two studies have been published that validate her remarks. One, a University of Wisconsin–Madison study published in the journal Toxicology and Industrial Health, *January-March 1999, found that the pesticide-fertilizer mixtures commonly found in groundwater can affect patterns of aggression and the ability to learn, and causes hormone disruptions that increase sensitivity to stimuli, irritability and immune dysfunction. A University of Arizona study published by* Environmental Health Perspectives *in June 1998 showed a decrease in mental ability and an increase in aggressive behavior among children exposed to pesticides.*

When I get exposed to chemicals I can't communicate, I can't speak, my brain shuts down, I can't translate the scattered thoughts into language. In school I got As and Bs without even looking at the books, but my high grades were never seen because of the impression that I gave. Quite often people thought that I was dumb.

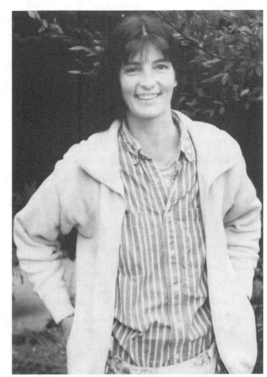

I see children now who look like I felt then. Their eyes are cloudy and they look dumb, and they look hyperkinetic when they get exposed to chemicals, or they get numb and comfy, kind of dazed.

As a child I often felt dizzy, or faint, and I'd squat down so I wouldn't fall over. I didn't know what it was at the time. I had severe headaches almost daily, and skin rashes. I used to get rashes all over my face, my arms, around my ears, the backs of my legs. The only thing that doctors could prescribe for me was a cortisone ointment that hurt and made my rash worse, so I didn't use it.

Being different, I was often alone. Instead of shying away from that I embraced that, even flaunted it. That was a coping skill. I've been that way my whole life. I feel fortunate. It's been lonely, but then, I guess pioneering is lonely. There have been times of wanting to be a pioneer and being proud of it, and times when I feel like I can't go on. Those feelings can be pretty heavy from time to time, when I'm not getting better or I feel I'm not getting anywhere by trying to raise awareness of environmental health issues.

An old friend of my parents introduced me to herbs when I was about six years old. It planted a seed in me that still grows. I actually began treating myself with herbs and vitamins when I was about fourteen. After high school I wanted to study alternative medicine, but I didn't want to go into a biology lab because the formaldehyde made me sick. So, instead of pursuing a college degree I wound up studying herbs on my own. Eventually I went to Montreal and studied with a woman there.

Ten years ago I came back to Victoria from Montreal with my firstborn, Nathan. I was twenty-six. I took another class in alternative health and herbs, and started working at the health food store here in town as an herbal consultant, ordering clerk and bookkeeper. I was in the process of putting together my own health food store—specializing in herbs and information, that sort of thing—when I became hypersensitive and more sick than I had been in my whole life. My nervous system, my brain, my kidneys shut down, and half my hair fell out.

It would have been easy for everybody in my family—and even me—to say I was crazy and write it off, if it hadn't been for Nathan. He developed asthma and had life-threatening episodes. It was through his reactions that I was able to get a view on my health, when I realized that we were getting sick at the same time. When I really started to pay attention, I saw a correlation between our episodes of illness and the timing of the military's firefighter trainings in this area. They were using diesel to start fires, and a toxic foam to put out the fires. A great, black cloud of smoke filled the air. At first I noticed that shortly after the burnings Nathan would develop a fever, diarrhea, and breathing difficulties, and I would be a nervous wreck. As time went on, we didn't seem to be reacting, but in reality our bodies were adapting. After that stage we reached the point where we were reacting immediately. Just to be sure of the correlation, I did some experimenting. I started taking us out of town during the burnings, and we got better. When we stayed in town for the burns, we got worse.

Nobody believed me except for one woman who came into the store a lot. She was so, so sensitive, and would have seizures with the burns. She also was so sensitive to pesticides that her skin burned from exposures she got just driving through the valley. Her mom drove her around trying to find a safe place for her, and they had to wrap her in a kind of material that helped to protect her from the pesticide exposures.

She and her mother and a friend of theirs were very helpful to me. They helped me to understand the development of allergies, chemical sensitivities, the spreading phenomenon, dietary needs, that type of thing. I don't know if I would have been able to do it on my own. For three years my children and I lived out of my truck during the burnings. Part of the time we stayed at a place up at Mt. Washington, where I felt dreadfully alone. No telephone. Very isolated. I was fearful most of the time. Terrified.

I found nontoxic paints and sealers to use in my house in Victoria and tore out the carpeting. One winter we went without heat because Nathan would have an asthma attack every time I turned it on. I wouldn't allow my mother to come over for almost a year because she always wore perfume and Nathan would have an asthma attack after she left. It took her a long time to understand. When my mom finally said to me, "Kate, I understand what you're telling me," after years of not understanding, it was a turning point for me. Then I could move ahead.

There have been some people in my life who I've had to stop seeing out of self-preservation. I may be lonely, but I'd rather be alone than have people around who will expose us to chemicals that make us ill.

My second child, Corey, will be five this year. He was born into a nontoxic household, so he hasn't been as sick. But after a pesticide exposure when he was fourteen months, he had a seizure and started banging his head. He'd have these tantrums and bang his head and scream because he was reacting, then scream because he was hurting himself and unable to stop.

I was thinking about the losses I have suffered from MCS, and a bumper sticker came to mind: "Of all the things I've lost, I miss my mind the most!" I absolutely feel like I've lost some of my mental abilities. It comes and goes. And when it's gone, it's really hard to notice, so I forgive people a lot in their not being able to recognize when it is happening to them. I look around, and I see people getting senile at thirty instead of seventy. They think it's normal. I think our potential is so much greater. I feel our general level of intelligence could be higher if it wasn't for the dumbing-down that we get from exposure to chemicals.

I believe, absolutely, that chemicals can alter our physiology, which can result in addictive behaviors, fear, even violence. There are chemicals that attack our nervous systems and affect our hormones, which changes our emotions and our ability to tolerate stress. So we can't take noise anymore, and we can't take the kids yelling, or three things happening at the same time. We blame our kids or the noise instead of blaming that which undermines our nervous system. We blame our fear on the crime rate, or whatever, instead of the chemically laced hot chocolate we drank or the pesticides we sprayed in the garden.

I cope with the fear by learning to recognize the cause and knowing that it will pass.

One of the things that has helped me the most is acknowledgment, and knowing that I'm not the only one with this illness. So many people have called me and said, "Oh, thank God! For years I thought it was just me!" Even though they're still sick and they don't know much about how to get better, they come away with greater strength, knowing they're not alone and the situation is real. That's probably one of the greatest coping mechanisms there is.

Where there is hope for everybody is in getting together. But it's very difficult for people who are chemically sensitive to get together. Shyness, insecurity, not being able to communicate—I see it in so many chemically sensitive people. At one point I took classes in modeling and acting to try to develop my self-confidence because, although I didn't realize the cause at the time, my reactions to chemicals had made me a very shy and withdrawn kind of person.

Talking about your chemical sensitivities can leave you vulnerable for abuse. Occasionally I've been attacked for my advocacy work. Last year my property was sprayed, accidentally or purposefully, with pesticides. I had kidney pain, hair loss and numbness for about three months. I did very little harvesting from my property, and many of my plants were damaged. It wasn't a normal pesticide application, it was a pesticide dump. So I'm way more sensitive to pesticides now than I was a year ago, and I'm very concerned about the spraying season coming up.

When I was working to stop aerial spraying in our area, I received a death threat. The purpose, of course, was to scare me and shut me up. And I was scared. But I figured that if I was going to die I'd better get out more information while I still could and I worked even harder.

Educating others is a major coping skill for me. I'm on the school board and have been working on policy development for about five years now. I've done a lot in that direction. As I see society recognizing the need for a cleaner environment, my hope is sustained. But, it's very slow work and frustrating. Maybe the information I deliver will be discussed, or maybe it'll go to a committee. When I hit a dead end, the anger builds. I'm learning how to communicate better and how to utilize anger without causing harm. Anger can be misdirected, especially when it can't be expressed directly to the people who are perpetuating disease without recognizing it. I use it to motivate me, in a way, to do something about the things I see. If I didn't have to keep going I would recede into being very quiet and unheard.

Those of us who do get out and get heard often make people angry. We're called crazy, and we might look crazy. Some of us are insecure and apologize a lot, or have antisocial behavior from chemical reactions or from the withdrawal from exposures.

I hope that by telling my story others will have hope that they can feel better. We can get better. We can create a safe environment for ourselves and our families, even if it is just a very small bit. We can set an example. It's okay to be different.

I'm concentrating on staying well, looking after my kids, and continuing with my life. New people are finally coming into my life, people who are on my wavelength.

Bernard Miller
Montreal, Quebec

A native of London, England, Bernard Miller lived and worked in twenty different nations over a period of thirty years. Travel and adventure shaped his life and work as an employee of the United Nations, the European Parliament and the European Union. In the following narrative he comments on the environmental health policies he has seen in action in various countries. Those comments are inspiring but bittersweet to me, because the U.S. compares so unfavorably.

As a child Bernard was allergic to cats, wool, chlorine, certain soaps and sunlight. He worked his way through architecture school in Great Britain by leading weekend tours throughout Europe. He studied city planning in Spain, developed a passion for issues related to housing policy and planning in developing countries, and eventually acquired a master's degree in urban development planning. He has worked on housing policy and elections in developing countries, and is fluent in eight languages.

Early in his career Bernard developed a "mystery" illness after a flu-like episode, and wound up seeing a series of doctors before the mystery was finally solved at the London Homeopathic Hospital. There he was diagnosed with an allergy to wheat. By eliminating wheat from his diet he enjoyed "perfect" health for almost a decade.

In 1990 he moved to Canada to work as an interpreter for a United Nations agency, hoping to pursue a doctoral degree in housing development at a nearby university. Within three weeks of his arrival he was ill from toxins in the building, although at first he didn't realize that was the cause. Eventually he learned that the building had been plagued with indoor air quality problems for years, and that allegedly the ventilation system was improved just before he came to work there. Largely due to Bernard's efforts some additional steps were taken to address the air quality problems. The agency approved and made Bernard coordinator of a Group for Action on Sick Building Syndrome Prevention (GASP), a working group which conducted a staff health survey and called for an independent air quality inspection of the building. Many problems were identified but never eliminated. Several employees collapsed while working in interpreting booths with poor air quality, and many suffered from sick building syndrome (SBS) before the agency moved out in 1996. Bernard learned the hard way that SBS can lead to full-blown MCS. He became completely disabled and in 1994 he was fired from his job on health grounds.

One of the losses Bernard experienced was his dream of earning a doctorate. After he was sensitized to chemicals the classrooms and library made him ill, his cognitive skills were impaired and chronic fatigue limited his activities.

I contacted Bernard when I heard he was looking for a safe place to stay in Seattle while attending a 1999 conference, and invited him to stay in my home. Together we attended the conference, "Chemicals, the Environment and Disease, A Research Perspective," sponsored by the University of Washington and the Washington State Department of Labor and Industry. For us, the highlight of the conference was when Howard Hu, a prominent Harvard researcher, physician and epidemiologist presented the results of his research on SPECT (Single Photon Emission Computed Tomography) Scans and MCS. Dr. Hu found that the blood flow in the brains of people with MCS is different from that of normal controls and from people

with chronic fatigue syndrome. Dr. Hu concluded that "These find-
ings are consistent with the hypothesis that MCS has a biological
basis and involves an alteration of function in the central nervous
system." Because this study will be peer-reviewed and cannot be
faulted for its methodology, it is a significant contribution toward
recognition of MCS in conventional medicine.

———————————————

When I was sixteen my father's cousin said to me, "You're young and idealistic and you'll grow out of it." Now I'm over three times that age and I'm much more idealistic and I'm definitely not growing out of it.

I want to spread the word about the dangers of environmental illness and about how easy it would be to prevent it. It's not a pipe dream. I've seen it. I want people to know the best of what's happening around the world, and not accept anything less—in terms of environment, health care, human rights and disability rights.

Come with me to Denmark and let me show you how medical research, worker protection laws, public opinion, consumer activism and cooperation right across the board have led to the removal of dangerous chemicals from the environment at every level. Come with me to Heidelberg, in Germany, and I'll show you a city that decided in the 1960s that it was going to be the most accessible city in the world for people with disabilities of all kinds. They've done that. Now they want to be the greenest city in the world, so they're competing with the city of Bologna to see which of them can produce the lowest level of emissions. I've seen it. I've been there. It's exciting.

The biggest fly in the ointment is the United States and the companies that own the United States. In Europe, people don't simply accept that business runs government. All across Europe there is a movement of people saying, "We won't buy food that is genetically modified." The European Union has said, "Label it or we won't let you sell it." Europeans won't buy meat containing carcinogenic hormones—that means U.S. meat. Canada has refused to buy a number of products from the United States—milk containing bovine growth hormones, for example. I, personally, wouldn't touch a dairy product produced in the U.S. unless it's guaranteed organic. In the U.S., industry dominates the government, meaning there is no labeling of genetically modified food and no possibility of consumer choice.

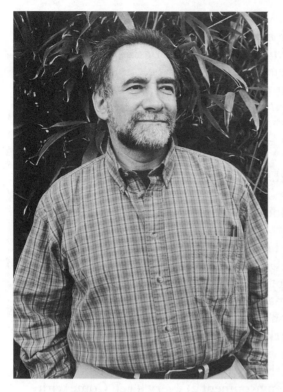

When I first got sick it didn't register with me what was happening. I thought maybe I was jet-lagged, although that had never happened to me before. I felt totally exhausted. I was getting headaches, and nosebleeds—which I'd never had before. I had difficulty concentrating. My eyes stung and turned bright red. I was dragging my feet. My hands and joints swelled. Nothing felt right. Then I'd go home and, within a hour, I'd start to feel better. Gradually I realized it was related to poor air quality, but I thought it was just a problem in *my* office. Then I learned that others in the building were experiencing symptoms, too, and colleagues told me people had been getting sick in the building for years. Within weeks I was falling asleep as soon as I got home from work. About midnight I'd wake up too tired to bother to eat. For a long time I'd been eating all organic, vegetarian, unprocessed foods. But I no longer had the strength to shop for or prepare whole foods. Nor did I have the strength to ride my bicycle. On the rare occasion when I did bike, I'd get partway down the canal I lived by and realize I couldn't carry on, so I'd have to chain up my bike and drag myself home to sleep.

When our environmental health working group was formed, we visited the print shop, located in the basement, and discovered there was no ventilation in that area. For fourteen years the printers had been working with toxic chemicals but no fresh air supply, and many of them were very ill. So the staff refused to work unless ventilation was installed in the print shop. The secretary general agreed to have the ventilation installed, making it the one place in the building to have adequate fresh air. It made me hopeful that we would get new ventilation throughout the building to make it a safe place to work.

We surveyed all the staff in the building to find out the nature and scope of health problems people were experiencing. Out of five hundred and fifty surveys circulated, four hundred and twenty-six were completed and returned. The results were phenomenal. Ninety-one percent of the respondents were experiencing classic sick building symptoms while they were in the building. But we were only surveying for immediate and short-term effects. What we didn't know was how many people who worked in the building since it opened in 1976 have since died of various cancers. I now know of at least thirty.

After the third collapse of an interpreter, in 1990, all meetings were moved to local hotels for three weeks. During that time eleven of us were sent to a physician for a histamine challenge test, which didn't produce any meaningful results, although the doctor did say we had symptoms compatible with sick building syndrome. I also went to see an allergist our workplace nurse had recommended. About two minutes into our meeting the doctor stopped me abruptly and said, "This sounds very much like sick building syndrome. I don't believe in sick building syndrome, I'm afraid I can't see you." That was the end of that visit.

By the end of my first year in Montreal the poor air quality was affecting so many people that meetings were stopped early two days in a row. The next morning conditions were even worse in the interpreting booths, so a message was sent to the president of the council of the organization, asking him to stop the meetings, which were due to end at one. Our request was ignored until five minutes to one, when the president announced, "I've received a message that we're having a little technical problem, so we are stopping the meeting early." I switched on my microphone and said, "The interpreters apologize. We do not have a little technical problem, we have a major health problem."

From that moment on all sorts of heavy-handed disciplinary measures were taken against me, all of which were illegal even within the UN, which doesn't offer much in the way of legal protection of staff. I was suspended from interpreting for most of the next year, which actually kept me out of the worst part of the building.

For six months I worked in Angola to help the UN supervise elections. While I was there I lived in a tent on a mountain, just on the edge of a rain forest, and my heath improved dramatically. But as soon as I went back to work in Montreal, my health deteriorated again within hours, just as if I had never been away from that building. It wasn't just me. A lot of the delegates from all over the world were complaining when they came to meetings. I was getting sicker and sicker.

I was aware of horrific fumes in the building. Even our nurse noticed them. So a colleague and I went up to have a look at the floor above us that was being renovated, and the fumes up there were unbearable. There were holes in the concrete slab directly above my desk—which I hadn't seen because my office had a suspended ceiling—and the fumes from upstairs were seeping through. I left the building and my doctor gave me orders to stay home for the next week. My boss tried to take disciplinary action against me. Later I learned that ten other employees had been sent home due to illness from the fumes the same day. No action was taken against them.

The UN wanted me to go to West Africa again for six months to organize elections in Guiné-Bissau and I thought things would be better when I returned. I still believed the agency intended to improve the air quality. So I accepted a new contract and sold my flat in London.

In Guiné-Bissau my health was much better, although not as good as it had been in Angola. When I started work again in Montreal after my return, I got so sick that I wrote a letter to the secretary general asking him what the agency was going to do to protect my health. Soon after that a meeting room was closed because of poor air quality, and I wrote again, saying I could no longer work there. That week the secretary general paid me $1,500 awarded by the UN tribunal for illegal disciplinary action taken against me two years earlier. Then he fired me, citing reasons of health and claiming that I was unable to fulfill my duties.

Official UN policy states that whenever an employee is dismissed on health grounds they have to propose a disability pension, but they did not do this for me. When I applied for disability benefit and compensation, the secretary general who fired me on health grounds claimed that I was not ill. To this day I am waiting for compensation. For five years I have been living on the proceeds from the sale of my flat, which have lasted longer than I anticipated. I expect I will run out of money sometime in the next year.

In addition to appealing through the UN's internal system, I have started a lawsuit against the building owner and the Canadian government. Two years on they are still challenging my right to sue, although two courts have upheld my right. My victory in the lower courts established an international point of law, the right of UN staff to sue their host government. Now the Canadian government is appealing to the supreme court.

When I was first fired I was stunned but relieved to be out of that building. I still thought that I would recover enough to be able to work in a safe environment. I wasn't concerned about money because I had the proceeds from the sale of my flat and I knew I could get work at the drop of a hat in Brussels and elsewhere. In fact, the Canadian government offered me work almost immediately. I still believed my health problems were limited to that one building. It took nearly a year before I fully realized how bad things really were. I was in great pain and having cognitive problems and severe fatigue. It took me several days to recover from one or two days of work in locations that had never bothered me before. At the time I didn't admit that I was too ill to work for other agencies, because I didn't want to burn any bridges.

I found myself spinning as fast as I could to take advantage of opportunities that came my way. But as soon as a door opened it was slammed shut in my face again because I couldn't do the work. My life became a nightmare. And eventually I had to cancel all contracts and refuse future work.

The hardest part for me is no longer having the ability to work on something from start to finish because of the cognitive problems I've developed. I'll start a project that should take me two hours, and three weeks later it still isn't finished. Once I got sick from exposures in a hotel and accidentally left my computer there and lost it. I've also lost a new camera and a wallet from putting them down and leaving them when I was having reactions.

I walk with a cane because I now have trouble with stairs and slopes, and when something moves across my visual field I can lose my balance and fall. There are days when I cannot get out of bed, I'm in such pain and so fatigued.

I've lost the ability to just *be*, without having to think about what might happen to me if I walk into a movie theater, or a library or a hotel. I have to worry about whether I might get trapped on the subway with somebody painting their fingernails, as happened to me once in London. I have to think before I do anything.

Occasionally I have fears about not being able to fend for myself, because I've had a few experiences that were terrifying. One happened when I was staying in a condo where I was exposed to fresh varathane. When I came out of the house it was snowing, and the movement of the snow across my visual field caused me to be totally disoriented. I didn't know where I was or where I was supposed to go. I actually sat down in the middle of the road, with cars driving around me, unable to think, until finally I came to and dragged myself off, but I was very sick for four days. I worry about something like that happening again. But I don't dwell on it.

I've also had the "charming" experience of becoming a nonperson. When I tried to use a credit card the authorization was denied because the card was issued to me as a staff member at the agency, and I was no longer a staff member. My health insurance was withdrawn by the agency. I was advised that my residency status was withdrawn by the Canadian government at the agency's request. And I had to apply to become an immigrant in order to stay in Canada and fight my case, but couldn't apply from within the country. So that was another year of hassles, but now I am officially an immigrant.

There was a period when I felt a lot of rage and other strong emotions, when all of a sudden I lost my job, my health care, my income, most of my friends, my home and my status in the country. After my dismissal I spent the first three or four years thinking my life was wasted. I still think that occasionally when I'm having a bad moment. But I try to use my anger creatively—by campaigning for environmental justice and civil rights, for example.

Interestingly, around the time that things got as bad as they possibly could—or at least that's what I thought at the time—I developed a more positive attitude. I found myself thanking God for anything even vaguely positive that occurred, such as beautiful skies or reflections of trees on water, or when I saw on the news stories of people who had endured difficulties that in the end turned out positive. I even found myself expressing gratitude for things like finding a lost pen or newspaper article. I felt especially hopeful when the first major settlements with the tobacco companies were made, and when the information they had covered up was revealed. Now I even give thanks when something seemingly negative occurs, on the basis that it is happening for a purpose. When I experience a delay, for example, I now see it as a gift of extra time to get more information or to meet a crucial new person or something like that.

Most friends and colleagues from work have not been very supportive. That's been difficult for me to accept. I didn't know anyone else who had the illness, except for people at work who were avoiding me because association with me after I was fired was considered dangerous. They thought being fired was contagious. Some friends have made well-intentioned suggestions, thinking they would be helpful—like telling me I ought to exercise more. They don't understand that my body won't let me exercise. My family doesn't understand MCS either.

The Internet was literally a lifesaver for me when I first realized I had MCS. Even now when I'm having a problem I get on the Internet and find somebody else who has had a similar experience. It's such a relief to have someone else who understands what I'm going through. And it helps me to share my experience and information with others. That way I don't feel totally useless.

I have just kept going. A lot of the time it has been entirely on my own. It's been tough, but I've become my own best friend. I'm glad I've got me twenty-four hours a day. I'm very comfortable with myself and I enjoy my company. That's a total transformation that's happened for me over the past five years. I really enjoy my solitude, but I also love being with other people.

What keeps me going is my conviction that if I keep on doing the right things, that right will triumph. Even though my appeal has not been decided yet, I believe I have won. I've got all the evidence. I have test results showing there are high levels of toxic chemicals in my fat tissue, and government studies showing the same chemicals found to be above acceptable levels in the building where I worked.

I'm happy with myself for doing what is right and for fighting against incredible odds for what I believe in. I can live with myself.

In the process of applying for disability benefits I was forced to see a doctor for an independent medical exam [IME]—which was anything but independent. This doctor asked me, "What do you think is your best characteristic?" I said, "My integrity." He said, "No, I mean a personality trait." I said, "My integrity." He said, "Behavioral—what are you good at?" I said, "Integrity."

A Voice
from Belarus

It is better to realize the truth through your own immediate experience than to accept without testing the teaching of another.—From *The Feminine Face of God* by Sherry Ruth Anderson and Patricia Hopkins

Anatoly Khramchenkov
Minsk, Belarus

A native of Russia, Anatoly Khramchenkov was raised in Belarus, a part of the former Soviet Union. He holds a Ph.D. in Germanic Languages from the University of Minsk, and currently is director of the foreign languages department of the Academy of Business Administration, started in Minsk in 1991 when Belarus became an independent state. He was a Fulbright scholar in business English and English as a second language.

After the nuclear explosion at Chernobyl in 1986, Anatoly and other professors and physicians created a foundation, For the Children of Chernobyl. Their goal was to send children abroad for the summers for a reprieve from radiation exposure which impairs their immune systems and has resulted in unprecedented levels of thyroid cancer in children and adults. The first host country to respond to their call for help was India. Before long, the foundation was sending 30,000 children every summer to host families and programs in many countries, including Germany, England, Japan, the U.S., Spain, Italy and France.

In summer 1997 my husband and I became a Children of Chernobyl host family. For me, it was a way to provide support to others with an environmental illness. The eight-year-old twin girls who lived with us that summer came from Belarus as part of a group chaperoned by Anatoly. During the third summer of hosting the twins, I inadvertently learned of Anatoly's adverse reactions to fragrances and other chemical exposures. We were on our way to a dental appointment for the girls, who spoke only Russian. While driving there, the girls mentioned to him that I was working on a book, and they wanted to know what it was about. Anatoly translated this to me, and when I explained to him that the book was about people with MCS, and explained the illness to him, he understood at once because of his firsthand experience of debilitating reactions to low-level chemical exposures. He explained to me that in his country unusual reactions to substances are all referred to as allergies, and that MCS is not yet in their vocabulary. Upon our arrival at the dental building we proceeded to the elevators where a few other people were also waiting. When the elevator arrived the others stepped in, one of them wearing a strong fragrance. Anatoly and I waited for the next elevator, both relieved to be in the company of someone who understood that decision without a single word of explanation.

The differences in environmental contaminants between our two countries are striking. In Belarus, "better living through chemicals" is not a lifestyle option. The economic crisis in the country is so devastating that most people can barely meet basic survival needs. Pesticides are not in heavy use, if used at all. New clothes are not affordable, let alone new carpeting. The use of preservatives, growth hormones and antibiotics in the production of food is almost unheard of. The majority of people don't own cars. On the other hand, in Belarus there are less restrictions on industrial pollution, there are no requirements for disclosure of ingredients in food and other products, and the food, air and water are contaminated by radiation pollution that will affect human health in untold ways for millenniums.

Despite our differences, some of the outcomes are undeniably similar: increased cancer rates and adverse reactions to ordinary products.

Over the years I have developed more and more allergies, and something strange happens to me when I am exposed to certain smells. It's like something in me opens up and I can smell almost anything so acutely, even objects that are far away from me. It's terrible. I mix up words or say something stupid. My face becomes red and my eyes tear.

Once, on a flight from London to Boston, there was a lady on the plane who was wearing some kind of deodorant with a scent that made me ill and gave me a horrendous headache. I felt so terrible that I could hardly move. She was sitting close to the front, and I couldn't even pass through that area to go to the bathroom because

I could smell this scent so acutely. This had never happened before, and I really felt embarrassed. That smell stayed with me for three or four days.

Another time I noticed something strange happening to me after my wife had used something to clean a spot on the upholstery of our sofa. I was lying there reading when suddenly the smell of the cleanser she had used became so strong, as if someone put it in my nose. Then I had a similar experience when my wife was doing laundry. The smell of the washing powder overwhelmed me. Now she can launder clothes only when I am not home, and I have asked her to please wear a mask whenever she is using washing powder, so that, hopefully, she won't also develop this allergy.

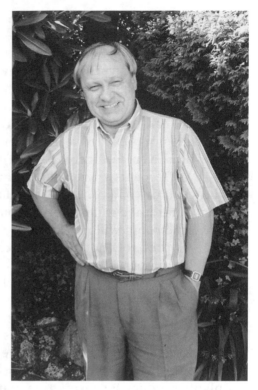

In our country we are not told the contents of any products, not even foods. When the democratic process started, the Ministry for Antitrust thought we should have disclosure of product ingredients so that people could supervise the quality of goods, especially the quality of food. But then, you see, the political situation changed drastically, so that ministry was banned. We don't know what we're using or eating. I can't drink milk in Belarus, because it's not really milk. It's a white, watery liquid with a horrible stinking smell.

I've also become very allergic to different kinds of paints. Some people were remodeling their apartment, and the fumes made me extremely ill. I could smell it fifty or one hundred meters away. It feels as though the smell gets into my lungs and head. It's a terrible feeling. Even after I'm standing a long time in the fresh air, in the open, I still have that smell.

When this kind of thing happens to me in the classroom while I'm teaching, I need to leave the room. I apologize to my students. I say, "Please don't pay attention; it's not my fault." I go to my study and open the window to bring in some fresh air. When it is over, I am okay. Everyone knows I have this condition. My wife knows. My son knows. My students know.

In our country it is hard to buy good perfume. So, when the girls buy perfume that is good—French made, not something fake—they want to put on as much as possible to show that they have it, you know. I had to explain to my students, in a not very sensitive way, that it is not polite to wear a lot of perfume, and that in some countries it is even considered vulgar.

My students are very understanding. They understand that even the smell of chalk in the classroom makes me sick. I bring special chalk and leave it in the classroom so that my colleagues who use the same room will not write on the blackboard with toxic chalk. Ours is probably not as pure as chalk in the United States.

I'd rather walk than take public transport, because when I am on a bus that is packed, I can smell everything and my life is terrible. I will ride for one or two or three stops, and when my life becomes unbearable and I cannot stay on the bus any longer, I simply get off and walk or wait for another bus that's not so crowded.

I think that I started to develop all of these allergies when I moved to Minsk. In the neighborhood where we lived there were plants producing construction materials. Whenever we opened the window there was black dust. There is also a lot of dust because the soil is sandy. When the municipal authorities had the money they sent out special trucks every night to wash the roads. But now they don't have the money, so there is a lot of sand on the roads.

I noticed that I became very allergic to dust. It was hard to breathe, and I got red spots on my nose and face, my eyes were watering and itching. It became worse and worse.

Before moving to Minsk I lived in a very small town with beautiful trees, and it was not as dusty. It was not an industrial city. That's why the air was much better. In Minsk there are a lot of industrial plants and pollution. I cannot go to certain areas because the smell would suffocate me, especially when it's hot. I cannot even imagine how people can work in those terrible conditions where they manufacture paint and other products.

You never know what might happen to you. The day of the explosion at Chernobyl, the sun was shining and it was a wonderful day. Who would suspect this would happen? Of course, we didn't know anything. I found out from a friend who knew someone who worked for the International Atomic Energy agency in Vienna. He called my friend and said, "Something terrible happened there, because the level of radiation has grown. We don't know what it is." My friend knew that my wife and two-year-old son were staying out in the country at her mother's. He called and told me to go there and bring my son and wife back to Minsk, and to keep the doors and windows closed. So I immediately took a train and brought my wife and child to Minsk. It was three days later that Mikhail Gorbachev admitted publicly that something terrible had happened. The radiation had reached Sweden, Norway, Finland and some other European countries, so he had no other choice. He couldn't keep all this information secret any longer. If he had warned the population that the explosion had taken place at Chernobyl, many lives could have been saved because every family has got iodine. A glass of water with one or two drops of iodine could have protected people. Their thyroids would have absorbed the iodine, which would have blocked the radioactive iodine. When the level of radiation was high, thyroids—especially kids' thyroids, because kids are so susceptible—absorbed a lot of radioactive iodine. And now we're having an unprecedented level of thyroid cancer. Several of my colleagues have died of thyroid cancer.

Two years ago when I was in the United States I had part of my thyroid removed because I had a tumor. After the surgery I was supposed to swallow a pain pill, but I couldn't do it. Not because it was painful for me to swallow. No, because I couldn't stand the smell of the tablet. I said, "Please, no! This smell kills me! I'd rather have the pain!"

The explosion at Chernobyl started a chain reaction. It's forever. You cannot stop it. The half-lives of various radioactive elements are different. The half-life of plutonium is twenty-four or twenty-five thousand years. We don't know how all of the radioactive elements affect our health, and there is mutation of different radioactive elements that have not been studied. To study this you need a lot of money.

A kind of shelter was built around the Chernobyl nuclear block after it exploded. It was okay for some time, but then huge cracks developed. It still spews radiation, which comes through all the cracks. On certain days you can feel it. Anyone can tell you when there was another spew of radiation, because you feel dizzy or you get a headache. One of my students had family who lived near Chernobyl, and whenever he went there to visit them it was like a nightmare for him. He said, "I'm very passive. I cannot do anything. I have no strength." A lot of kids have those symptoms from radiation exposure.

Every spring when the farmers start plowing, all the radiation absorbed by the soil gets turned up. The moment the wind starts blowing it spreads very quickly. No one will ever know the truth about how many people have become sick or died from radiation exposure, because there was some special regulation so the doctors have no right to disclose this information. If someone died of radiation, the diagnosis was something different.

The majority of people who took part in the cleanup operations were soldiers. They came from different parts of the former Soviet Union, from different villages. How can you trace what has happened to them? No one asked them if they wanted to go or not. It was an order. They were young boys. I have seen documentaries showing them standing on the roof of that reactor, wearing nothing but their uniforms. Some were given lead aprons to wear, but those don't protect the whole body. I think the majority of them who went there have died or they're now invalids. Those who survived don't want to marry because they don't want to be responsible for bringing children with abnormalities into the world. We have so many children with abnormalities now. They will never be able to prove it is from the radiation. You cannot touch it. You cannot feel it. How can you prove it?

All of Belarus was contaminated. But the only people who are monitored for the effects of radiation, and who receive vitamins and medicines and humanitarian aid, are those who were directly involved in the cleanup or who lived in the area now known as the Dead Zone. All the others, no one cares what happens to them. They aren't even monitored. So kids are dying. They are taken to hospital when it's too late because no one monitors them.

Because of Chernobyl many people's immune systems are so weak that people are more susceptible to allergies. There is a special center in Minsk for people with allergies. They try to find some kind of medication, but medication is so expensive now that you cannot afford to buy it. If you don't take any medication, you can suffocate. What other sicknesses we might have, or might develop in the future, no one knows.

When my son, Vitaly, was a small boy we couldn't take him anywhere because he would get sick and vomit on a bus or in a car.

At the time it was diagnosed as motion sickness, but in fact it was not motion sickness. He couldn't stand the smell of gas. Our cars and buses burn diesel, and no one cares about the amount of emissions. There are black clouds of exhaust fumes everywhere.

This year, in the United States, he was invited to go on a trip to Montana. He probably wanted to go. He refused. I think it was because he knew he would feel sick on the long drive, but I don't ask because I know he feels embarrassed.

In this life anything might happen to you. I think we should create an atmosphere of awareness regarding environmental health issues, before it is too late.

A Significant Other Voice

The stories people tell have a way of taking care of them. If stories come to you, care for them. And learn to give them away where they are needed. Sometimes a person needs a story more than food to stay alive. That is why we put these stories in each other's memory. This is how people care for themselves.—From Crow and Weasel *by Barry Lopez*

Curt Schuster
Detroit, Michigan

Chronic illness affects everyone in relationship with the person who is ill, particularly those who live together. Multiple chemical sensitivity affects other members of the household more profoundly, perhaps, than any other illness because of the many accommodations required. Many relationships don't survive stressors of this magnitude. In light of this, it seemed important to include in this book a narrative on coping from the viewpoint of a healthy person who loves and lives with someone who has MCS.

Interestingly to me, I found some spouses reluctant to discuss the effects of MCS on themselves or their marriage. To me this reflects the level of difficulty and complexity associated with their roles as partner, support person, and accommodator.

In the narrative that follows, Curt Schuster articulates some of the issues faced by spouses, and his style of coping. Although it wasn't planned, his wife Elizabeth was the first person interviewed for this collection and he was the last. In my opinion, I couldn't have chosen more appropriate "bookends."

I found Curt to be thoughtful and candid in his remarks. So much so that during the interview I realized a part of me was braced for hearing painful truths about living with a partner who has MCS, truths which might be unspoken or denied within the boundaries of an intimate relationship, including my own. What I found, however, was that his love and compassion for Elizabeth enabled me to hear his frustration and grief with empathy.

After the interview he expressed to me his gratitude for the opportunity to reflect on and characterize his experience of MCS. His expression of gratitude deepened my appreciation for the importance of recognizing and acknowledging the challenges, needs and triumphs of the unsung heroes who support those of us with MCS.

    Curt is the general manager of a large landscape company and nursery. His policy is to avoid the use of pesticides, although there are rare occasions when he will resort to using them at work. On those occasions he hires professional applicators and leaves the area to minimize his own exposures and to reduce the risk of bringing home residue that would impact Elizabeth.

    Curt enjoys physical labor and working outdoors. He shares with Elizabeth an interest in Buddhism and meditation. They are celebrating twenty-five years of marriage this year with a trip to St. Thomas Island, where they have reserved a small stone castle overlooking the Caribbean.

I value this relationship so much that it's a natural thing for me to accept MCS as a part of it. I'm not leaving this relationship, so I accept that this is how it is. This is one of the parameters of this relationship that I, as a spouse, have to deal with. The MCS is not going to go away. This is a part of our life. By accepting that, it's a whole lot easier to move through all of the problems it presents. The Buddhist idea of acceptance is helpful to me.

Elizabeth is a brilliant woman with a great career. She's done incredible work on herself in a spiritual sense and psychological sense. She has all these positive qualities, and she has to deal with MCS all the time. It's a daily thing. What makes me most angry is how difficult it makes her life, and how MCS affects her quality of life. She has to plan how she goes about her life in relation to how her environment is going to affect how she feels. As a result of that, I have also become hypervigilant.

The average couple walking in a mall to shop is literally not giving a thought to their environment. Whereas *everywhere* we go I'm instantly hypersensitive to the environment. Every time we walk into a shop or restaurant I'm wondering: Is Elizabeth going to be able to handle this? That's pretty much second nature now. There's always a little bit of apprehension.

I tend to look at situations as just problems to be solved. When Elizabeth experienced her first major chemical reaction ten years ago, I saw it as just something to deal with. It's hard for me to remember what my frame of mind was then. I don't think I made any assumptions about it. I didn't think in terms of a chronic illness. I just thought this is what we're dealing with now. As it escalated and we became a little more educated and realized it wasn't going to go away, I felt all the normal feelings: anger, grief, frustration.

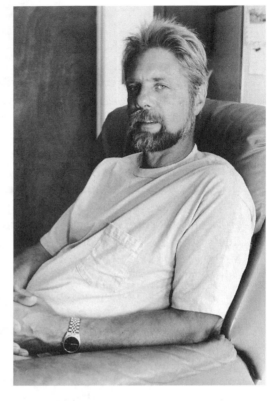

It was a real crisis point after we bought this house and realized it wasn't safe for her. It was physically and emotionally overwhelming for her. For me it was, okay, this is serious, so how are we going to deal with it? It wasn't my health that was at risk.

A key question for the spouse of someone with MCS is: Are you willing to let go of control of your environment? Because the person suffering with MCS has to take aggressive control of their environment. But in order for them to do that, the spouse has to relinquish control almost one hundred percent. You have to learn to surrender. I don't mean surrender in the sense of losing the battle. I mean it in a more spiritual sense, where you surrender certain aspects of your life on behalf of somebody else. It's a conscious surrender on behalf of the relationship. It's a flat-out giving on the spouse's part. It's one-sided. It's a simple concept, but it's really difficult to do. You have to accept that this is your situation. You can't think you're going to change it, because you're powerless. Believe me, I'm not saying this is easy. I'm not talking degree of difficulty. I'm just saying this is what works for me. If you can't accept it, then either the relationship is not going to last or you're going to go nuts.

Any life has problems. Any relationship has problems. If your spouse comes down with a medically recognized chronic illness, dealing with chronic medical problems becomes a part of the relationship that requires a change in how you approach the relationship. MCS presents the same kinds of issues as any chronic illness, and requires different sacrifices by the spouse.

In many ways Elizabeth is incredibly healthy. I'm always confident that she's going to bounce back from a chemical reaction, that it's not going to be permanent. Sometimes when she has a horrible brain reaction, she's afraid she might permanently lose some of her mental faculties. I never feel that way. No matter how exposed or how sick she is, I always believe that it will pass. It's not that I'm in denial. She has a core constitution that is really strong. That's something she has to be reminded of sometimes.

When she is really having a tough time and really brain-fogged from an exposure, it affects her emotionally. And one of the ways she deals with it is to withdraw. She doesn't have the energy to give to a spouse. She's taking care of herself. She just tries to hang on. That's a loss.

There are also material losses. MCS has a real impact on the material settings of your life. I think the reason that part has not been difficult for me is that we're not real materially oriented to begin with. We're not avid consumers. If I was the type of guy who got upset because I can't have a new car or a lot of furniture, or because we can't paint the walls every two years, then I would have problems. But I don't care about that stuff. That's not to say that we wouldn't have some different things than we have, given the choice.

We've really altered how we live. For example, we sleep in the living room because it's safe for Elizabeth; we have for five years. That doesn't provide a whole lot of privacy, but I'm so used to it that it would seem kind of weird to start sleeping in a bedroom with a door closed.

The material goods we have tend to be old and inert. This glass dining room table is not something we would choose as a style, but it's safe. For us, it is a great replacement for the old table we had before this. This is a victory. That's how I look at it.

Quite frankly, I'm amazed that we have this air conditioner. It's a small quality of life thing, but it works and I love it. We bought this last week and I figured that I would have to cover it up with aluminum foil, that it wouldn't be safe.

When we moved into this house there was linoleum on the kitchen floor that made Elizabeth sick. We'd used up most of our money to move into this house, but we had to have that linoleum torn out. Then I put in a hardwood floor—which was hard work—and *that* didn't work. So then I hired some guys to put in this ceramic tile.

The whole lower section of the house was carpeted, and there were molds in the carpet. So I tore all of that out and put in ceramic tile. Would we have chosen ceramic tile for most of the house? Probably not. But I like it now that I'm used to it.

When I buy new clothes I know I won't be able to wear them around Elizabeth for a while, because that's one of the things that makes her sick. I actually feel worse for her because it's so hard for her to find clothing she can wear. One out of twenty pieces of clothing is safe for her. All the clothes we buy are made of natural fibers so the level of toxicity is lower.

Automobiles are a real hassle. Because of Elizabeth's reactions to products used in cars, my choices in automobiles are narrowed down by about ninety-nine percent. So we try to find cars that will satisfy some of my desires and still work for her. An old Mercedes-Benz meets both of our needs, although the one we just purchased isn't working for us yet because it smells of fragrances worn by the previous owners. We're hoping it will off-gas.

Vacations are difficult. We know going into it that the whole trip could be a disaster. We take precautions to try to ensure that there's as little toxicity as we can plan for. But we can never plan for all of it.

We took a trip to Oregon last summer. Three of the four places where we made advance reservations worked out fabulously. One was horrible. We were in the middle of a ten-day vacation. Everything was going along great until we got to this place. At first Elizabeth tried to ignore that she was having a chemical reaction; she sometimes copes, initially, with some denial. Two or three hours later she finally gave in to the reality of it. I knew she was feeling like hell. The only room in the whole place that she could tolerate was the bathroom. It was a nightmare. What were we going to do? It was late at night. Was she going to sleep on the front lawn? in the bathtub? I was shuffling back and forth between her and my son, trying to take care of both of them. She's emotionally vulnerable at those times, and she was worried about the effect her reaction would have on the family and our vacation. Our son was worried about his mom and wondering what was going on, although he seems to handle these situations very well and understands what we tell him about it.

By three in the morning I was exhausted. It was a horrible night. I was up all night, not knowing how Elizabeth was going to be. Was she going to be in a brain fog for the rest of the vacation? But in those situations I have to take care of them first and then try to take care of myself. It's not a time that I can express how I'm feeling, when she's feeling physically bad and mentally disoriented and emotionally flayed from chemical exposures.

The next day we drove on down the coast and found a bed and breakfast that was safe, and it was five times nicer than the place we'd been. Elizabeth's head was cleared somewhat. She was still achy, but we were a family unit back on vacation and it was cool.

I tend to believe that's what's going to happen, somehow, most of the time. I can't think of too many situations where it doesn't work out that way. I'm better than I used to be at just accepting those situations. I'm not going to say I'm so enlightened that I can meditate it away. That doesn't work. Sometimes I get mopey, but not for very long. Or I get pissed off. I kick it around internally. But I don't brood over it. I'll go out for a walk and tell myself, okay, this is what we're doing, get a grip here. But in the moment when something like that is happening its hard to keep a grasp on it.

These are our problems to deal with. It doesn't matter about anybody else. I had a real revelation about that five years ago when we leased a new van for two years. We thought it would only take a couple of weeks to air out before it would be okay for Elizabeth. But we were wrong. It was horrible. In January we were driving around with all the windows down. I tried really hard to get Ford Motor Company to let me out of that lease. I explained the situation and made a real issue about it—we'd barely put any miles on the van and I was willing to pay a premium to get out. When they still wouldn't let me out of the lease I ranted and raved about how I'd bought Ford cars for twenty-five years and how my father had worked for Ford. Finally, after about a week of this, I woke up one morning and thought to myself, you know, this isn't Ford Motor Company's problem. It's your problem. What are you getting mad at them for? They've fulfilled their part of the agreement.

It wasn't anybody's problem but mine, and I needed to be a little more creative about what we were going to do about it. That was kind of a breakthrough for me. It helped me. We ended up asking my dad if he wanted a new van for two years, and he traded us for his old station wagon. It worked out fine.

Elizabeth doesn't ask a lot. The condition asks a lot of us as a family unit. What it boils down to is, I choose to do these things. The whole thing is real simple. Either you love your spouse enough and the relationship has enough value to you that you don't really question what you have to do. You just do what you have to do. That's how it is.

The emotional aspect is the hardest part for a spouse, in my opinion. The difficulty for us is keeping an open line of communication without adding to each other's burden. That's a hard line for me to tread. When her condition is getting me down I can't turn to her like I do with everything else in my life. She may be the source of my stress or anger or frustration, but not the cause of it. She has enough to deal with. She doesn't need me to be unloading how I'm feeling about it. That's difficult because we share everything else.

I don't want it to sound as if I'm protecting her. I'm not. One of the reasons we've been married so long is because we have a real open line of communication and we're honest with each other and try to deal with everything out in the open. We try to be emotionally honest with each other. But it's difficult to discuss with her how I am feeling about her condition, or how it affects me. Those discussions are difficult. We still haven't fully developed a language that works for us.

At the risk of sounding like I have a really high opinion of myself as a spouse, I feel I'm incredibly supportive. I don't think there's a whole lot more I could do. I'm supportive of any course of treatment Elizabeth is interested in exploring. When she asks me what I think about a treatment modality, my response has always been that if it's something that she thinks might work or will have some positive benefit, then I'm for it.

There are some things we would probably do more if Elizabeth didn't suffer from MCS. We'd go to more social functions and live performances. Elizabeth dislikes wearing a mask in public, but it doesn't bother me. That's easy for me to say because it's not me. Quite honestly, I don't really care very much what other people think about us—although I admit that there's a part of me that sometimes wishes we didn't have to deal with an illness that isn't recognized or understood. When we do go out for an evening there's always a chance that a person sitting near us will be wearing so much fragrance that even *I'll* be gagging. We hope for the best.

Elizabeth and I have a really great relationship. Being able to forge a strong relationship around chronic illness has contributed to that. We believe that we can choose to learn and grow from events that happen in our lives. Problems and heartaches and chronic conditions enable us to learn more about ourselves. All I can say is that it works real well for us. God knows I wish the MCS was gone. It's horrible. But it is here and these are some of the ways we have benefited by going through this.

Appendix A:
A Sociologist's View

Steve Kroll-Smith, Ph.D.
Research Professor of Sociology
University of New Orleans

Steve Kroll-Smith studies people affected by dangerous or extreme environments. More specifically, he's interested in how people cope when, due to lack of information and support, they are left to their own devices to understand and respond to environmental crises. He has studied people who live in Super Fund communities; residents of Centralia, Pennsylvania, a town where a mine fire raged underground; and people with multiple chemical sensitivities.

Steve first heard of MCS from a woman he met at a conference, a former Environmental Protection Agency employee who was disabled by chemical exposures in her workplace. Intrigued by her story, he called the Louisiana Environmental Action League in Baton Rouge. The agency confirmed that they were receiving calls in growing numbers from workers who, following an initial chemical insult on the job, had become sensitized to many substances, and were experiencing reactions that "should not be happening." For further information he was referred to Diane Hamilton, a former chemist with MCS who facilitates a support group in Baton Rouge, and whose story appears in this book. Diane invited him to attend a meeting of the group. He went, and was intrigued by the stories that he heard. Over the next five years he studied issues related to MCS. Out of that work came a book he co-authored with H. Hugh Floyd, Bodies in Protest: Environmental Illness and the Struggle Over Medical Knowledge *(New York University Press, 1998).*

Steve does not have MCS. He makes the following observations based on his interactions with the many chemically ill people he interviewed while researching for his book.

———————————

I've always thought of the body as something you approach as a thing to know; but now I'm much more prepared to believe that the body itself is a way of knowing. I've been challenged by this work because it's taken me in the direction of looking at the body as a source of knowledge.

Why should we not believe that bodies change in relationship to changed environments? We have reason to believe MCS is more than likely an indicator of this kind of change. We may, in fact, have a new body amongst us, a body that is less tolerant to invasive chemical exposure, that is asking for change in a visceral kind of way.

I found this idea very interesting as a public health issue. So I decided that I would start interviewing people who are environmentally ill. The people I interviewed included orchestra conductors, plumbers, accountants, chemists and painters.

As a social psychologist, I was struck by how strong people were in managing this illness—or how weak they were in managing this illness—in relationship to the other people in their lives. The people who seemed to cope the best with this illness were those who had a strong social network, who had other people who will listen to them and who will empathize with them and will make some changes in their own lives so that they can continue in relationship with them. If there is a social space you can set up in such a way to help you manage this chronic illness, you're leagues ahead of others, and possibly will be able to adapt. Those who seem to adapt well are those who recognize they're going to have to renegotiate their social space. You're going to have people in your social world who are accommodating because they like you and respect you; they're going to make the changes. You've got people who aren't going to do that. Part of the coping process becomes admitting there are people who you thought were close, who aren't going to understand. To survive you've got to say good-bye to those people in one way, shape, or form. This changing and realignment of social space is, I think, a necessary part of adaptation.

With married couples, there's a big difference between those where the spouse said, "I can't understand what's going on with you, I can't get on board with you," and those who said, "I'm here to help you." Intimate others who accept the illness are extraordinarily helpful. Close friendship networks are extraordinarily helpful—even if it's one other person you can talk to. This illness isn't something you can do by yourself.

I met a lot of people who, prior to MCS, would say yes to everything that was asked of them. Now they're much more judgmental of the things they do and don't do, and feel they have a little more control over their lives. I think that's necessary for healthy coping.

Probably the most powerful coping technique for folks with environmental illness is similar to the coping techniques for people in trauma. That is to have some control over your own emotional response. Some have a real visceral chemical reaction that affects their emotions, I understand that. But to be empowered in some way, to make decisions on your own behalf, to take some responsibility for shaping the world you live in—it works. To take charge of what you can do, even if it's a small thing to make your life just a little bit better.

Anger is a necessary part of making the adjustment, of grieving over a lost way of life. But anger shouldn't capture the self. When it becomes an obsession, that's when it diminishes your capacity to act on your world. Then it becomes an extraordinarily tiring experience. And if you've already got an immune system that's not what it should be, chronic anger is simply going to amplify the problem.

Another coping strategy I saw was helping other people. Those people who have reached a point where they can help other people, that has pushed them over the top in their healing.

Something that impressed me about the people I interviewed is how proactive and involved they are in doing something about their illness. They wouldn't be spending that kind of money and time on different treatments, or making extraordinary sacrifices to find a safe place to live, if they just wanted people to feel sorry for them. They are able to identify what's wrong and, while they can't cure themselves, they are able to make themselves somewhat better by avoiding chemical exposures and making lifestyle and diet changes. They end up better off than when they were seeing a series of docs. In other words, the treatment regimen, while certainly not curative, works for many people. I'd have every reason to believe in that myself;

every reason to believe in that. The fact that biomedicine can't explain these things doesn't mean it's not biomedical. Biomedicine has a terribly difficult time with etiology.

Disease is political. It's always been political. The idea that the medical profession sees something, recognizes it as a disease and puts it on the books is false. That's not how it happens. You struggle to get these things recognized.

Look at asbestosis. Look at the fight that had to go on to recognize asbestosis, which is clearly much more visible and much more particular, with a particular body system that is affected by a particular agent. That should be pretty simple to figure out, but it took how much grassroots action, how much legislative tweaking? Finally it was recognized.

This is a particularly high-stakes struggle because, if environmental illness is recognized, we're going to have to rethink the way we consume things. And that's a major shift. There's a lot at stake there. A lot of stakeholders.

What will happen is, there will be a successful court case in which environmental illness gets put on the books as a diagnosis. It's not going to be the medical profession that does it. The legal profession will push the medical profession into recognizing it. That's the model for creating disease in this society. So don't look for some researcher in some biomedical lab somewhere to say, "I found it!" What'll happen is somebody will be lucky enough to get their case heard and get it on the books and it will be recognized in that fashion. Mary Lamielle, in New Jersey, has testified in front of Senate subcommittees on environment and health and she's gotten the definition of environmental illness into congressional records. So it's there.

It's a dangerous illness, politically, because it demands so much change. It's different enough that it's easy for some people to move it from the body to the mind. I hope my book is a corrective to some of the critics that are too ready to write this illness off as neurotic somatization. They're too ready to move it from the body to the mind. Environmental illness doesn't fit any of the hysterical contagion models that are out there, and there aren't any real secondary gains associated with this illness.

This illness is going to be recognized. There are a number of medical academics and researchers with prestigious appointments who validate this illness. Nicholas Ashford and Claudia Miller have published a very straightforward account of MCS in their book

[*Chemical Exposures: Low Levels and High Stakes, Second Edition* (New York: John Wiley & Sons, 1998)]. He's an attorney and an engineer at MIT. Claudia Miller is a physician at the University of Texas. They're both high-profile professionals. We'd be remiss not to take them seriously. They point out in their book this illness cuts across demographic groups, it cuts across economic class, it cuts across race, it cuts across gender.

Something I found striking is that a number of organizations and institutions—certainly not an adequate number—are willing to recognize MCS and to make accommodations. I find it interesting that this is going on simultaneously with almost studied denial of MCS, as an environmental illness, on the part of the mainstream medical profession. That's a kind of institutional learning I'm not accustomed to seeing. But there are changes taking place independent of an affirmation by the American Medical Association.

Some changes are being made through the courts. The Americans with Disabilities Act is being used successfully to get some changes made at the workplace. Marin County, California, has established a fragrance-free zone in the county courthouse. The Berkeley library is fragrance-free. The Minnesota School of Social Work is scent-free. HUD has said that for every twenty units of public housing that are built, one unit has to be fitted for the environmentally ill. Social Security will consider chemically related illness claims, on a case-by-case basis. Canada has put some money into research on MCS and is beginning to recognize it with policy. The state of Maryland has been a little more progressive than other states, and New Mexico has become more aggressive.

So these changes are going on. Multiple chemical sensitivity will get recognized. It's happening now.

Appendix B:
What Is Multiple
Chemical Sensitivity?

*A part of the following overview is adapted from the book-
let,* Multiple Chemical Sensitivity.[1] *For in-depth information on
the physical and medical aspects of MCS and theories of cau-
sation, please refer to books recommended in Appendix C and
Appendix D.*

Scientists acknowledge that many substances contain chemicals
known to be toxic in high concentrations. To chemically sensitive
people, these and other substances can be harmful even in minute
amounts. A whiff of hair spray, fresh paint or bug spray, for example, can be debilitating to a person with multiple chemical sensitivities. People with MCS must avoid chemical exposures or symptoms
will persist or worsen and the illness will progress.

The exact mechanism by which chemical exposures cause MCS
is unknown. It is believed that a two-step process occurs. First, an
initial exposure or chronic exposures interacts with a susceptible
individual, leading to loss of that person's prior, natural tolerance
for everyday, low-level chemicals, as well as certain foods, drugs,
alcohol, and caffeine. In the second stage, symptoms are thereafter
triggered by extremely low doses of previously tolerated products
and exposures.[2] This theory is called toxicant-induced loss of tolerance or "TILT."[3]

Pesticides and solvents are the two classes of chemicals most
frequently identified as having initiated the illness. Some people
develop MCS after a single major exposure, like an industrial accident, while others become sick seemingly as the result of the cumu-

lative exposures of daily life. Some people can pinpoint the exact chemical exposure that led to their chemical sensitization, while others have no way of knowing what made them ill. One particularly dangerous and frequently hidden source of chemical exposure is the common practice of applying pesticides to apartment complexes, restaurants, schools, hospitals and other public and private buildings without notifying the occupants.

Researchers speculate that in MCS certain chemicals damage the nervous system, particularly the area of the brain called the limbic system. Neurological damage might explain a broad range of chemical reactions in people with MCS, from stomach pain, urological problems and respiratory disorders to cognitive abnormalities and mood disorders, because the brain controls functions throughout the body.

Chemicals may also damage the immune system and enzymes that are required to detoxify harmful substances. It is also speculated that MCS symptoms may be caused by impaired blood circulation or the body's decreased ability to extract or use oxygen from the bloodstream. Lead, mercury and other heavy metal exposures can contribute to the development or aggravation of MCS as well.

It is likely that some or all of these mechanisms are involved in chemical sensitivity, and that disease occurs when the "total load" of biological, chemical, physical and psychological stressors exceeds a critical threshold for any particular individual. When the body is burdened by multiple stressors, susceptibility to MCS as well as other diseases is increased. It is not uncommon for trauma to precede or exacerbate this illness.

What Kind of Reactions Do People with MCS Experience?

Almost any symptom can occur in chemically sensitive people. The unifying factor in people with MCS is that their symptoms come and go in relation to chemical exposures that do not ordinarily affect others. The symptoms are diverse and unique to each person. The same chemical exposure may trigger different symptoms or none at all in different individuals. Usually more than one body system is affected and frequently involves the brain and central nervous system. Some common symptoms are headache, fatigue, sleep disturbances, asthma and other respiratory problems, gastrointestinal problems, impaired circulation, arthritis, joint and muscle pain, chest pain and heart irregularities, swelling, throat closing, burning sensations, weakness, depression and other affective problems, concentration and memory problems, learning impairment, difficulty thinking and speaking, and seizures. Food intolerance is also common and may be so severe that a person's diet is limited to only a few foods.

While many of the symptoms reported by people with MCS are similar to known toxic reactions, they usually occur at exposure levels previously thought to be safe. Additionally, many chemically sensitive people experience symptoms vastly different from typical toxic reactions.

Symptoms can range from mild to disabling and can even be life threatening. Reactions may vary depending upon the person's general state of health and the amount of other recent exposures. The onset of symptoms following an exposure may be immediate or delayed for hours or even days, and quite often are masked by the effects of ongoing exposures. Symptoms can last from a few seconds to a few weeks or months. Some people experience distinctly different constellations of symptoms in response to different substances. New symptoms may develop over time, and some may resolve. People with moderate to severe cases of MCS may be partially or totally disabled for several years or for life. Many improve but full recovery is rare.

Children with MCS may have red cheeks and ears, dark circles under their eyes, learning disabilities and behavior problems as well as other symptoms.

What Products Will Trigger an Adverse Reaction in People with MCS?

Substances that frequently cause symptoms in chemically sensitive people include pesticides, perfume, fresh paint, new carpets, many building materials, solvents, ink, smoke, vehicle exhaust, industrial fumes, plastics, petrochemicals, many cleaning products and scented products, including laundry soap, fabric softener, shampoo, hair spray, mousse, body soap, lotions, room deodorizers and aftershave. Naturally occurring chemicals such as tree sap and essential oils may also be problematic. Symptoms can occur after inhaling, touching or ingesting these or other substances. In addition, people with MCS may be sensitive to electromagnetic fields (EMFs).

Is MCS an Allergy?

Because people with MCS react to chemicals at levels that ordinarily do not affect others, chemical sensitivity is sometimes referred to as chemical "allergy," although the mechanism is not the same as in the more traditional allergies. A person with MCS may react to animals, pollen, dust and mold with symptoms that are the same or different from those of traditional allergies. People with MCS may also have common allergy symptoms such as itchy eyes, nasal congestion, sinusitis, asthma, hives and other rashes that result from exposures to chemicals or typical allergens.

Is MCS Related to Other Illnesses?

Frequently, MCS involves imbalances in one's nervous, immune, and endocrine systems, and impaired detoxification abilities. Conditions such as CFIDS (Chronic Fatigue Immune Dysfunction Syndrome), fibromyalgia, and Candida Syndrome are frequently found in people with MCS. It is not yet known whether these are separate diseases or whether they represent different manifestations of a common underlying problem.

Chemical exposures may play a role in causing or exacerbating many other chronic illnesses including depression, headaches, arthritis and asthma, and can cause cancer.

The most recent SPECT scan (single photon computed tomography of the brain) studies, by a Harvard School of Public Health physician and researcher, have shown that people with MCS have blood flow patterns in the brain that are different from those of healthy controls and from people with Chronic Fatigue Syndrome.[4]

Multiple chemical sensitivity is sometimes misdiagnosed as a psychiatric illness by physicians who do not recognize or understand this illness, and who are confused by the fact that people with MCS often experience emotional and psychological distress. However, these symptoms are frequently reactions to chemical exposures. For example, solvent exposures can precipitate panic disorders, depression and anger, and symptoms that mimic post-traumatic stress disorder.[5-8] Depression, anxiety and anger also are experienced as secondary reactions to the profound life changes and losses experienced by people with MCS. Unfortunately, there is insufficient help available for coping with the psychosocial impact.

Who Gets MCS?

Prevalence studies consistently indicate that 15 to 37 percent of the U.S. population report heightened sensitivity to chemicals. A large study done in California by the Department of Health Services revealed that 6 percent of the general population of California has been diagnosed with environmental illness, and over 16 percent of the general population reported an unusual sensitivity to common chemicals such as fragrances, cleaning products and garden sprays.[9] A New Mexico study revealed that 2 percent of the population in that state had been diagnosed with MCS, and over 2 percent had lost or left a job or career due to chemical sensitivities.[10] A 1998 study by the department of Veterans' Affairs found that MCS afflicts 36 percent of Gulf War veterans.

Multiple chemical sensitivity occurs in people of all ages, races and economic backgrounds, and is more prevalent in women than in men. Reports from around the globe indicate that MCS is a worldwide public health concern. Many people develop MCS after moving into a new home, working in a new or remodeled building, or after exposure to pesticides. High risk groups include students, teachers, office workers and others in tightly sealed buildings; residents in communities exposed to toxic waste sites, aerial pesticide spraying, groundwater contamination or industrial pollution; Gulf War veterans; infants, children, the elderly and people exposed to chemicals in their work.

Factors that may predispose one to MCS are a genetic predisposition, poor nutritional status, hormone imbalances, a history of trauma, and the presence of another illness or disability.

Anyone who is increasingly bothered by perfume or cigarette smoke or holds their breath when walking down the detergent aisle in a grocery store may be experiencing early signs of MCS. Having a history of unusual reactions to prescription or street drugs may also indicate that a person already has some degree of abnormal chemical reactivity.

How Long Has MCS Been Around?

Reports of heightened sensitivity to chemicals have been documented since the 1800s. Since World War II, there has been a dramatic rise in the manufacture and use of synthesized chemicals like pesticides, plastics, and artificial fragrances, and the incidence of MCS has steadily grown. One of the first doctors to identify the relationship between low-level chemical exposures and chronic illness was Theron Randolph in the 1950s.

Aren't Most Chemicals Tested for Safe Exposure Levels?

The full range of toxicity of most chemicals is not known, even chemicals used in fragrances and other personal care products. Few chemicals have been adequately studied for their effect on the nervous and immune systems. Little is known about the cumulative effects of chemical exposures. Even less is known about the effects of exposure to more than one chemical simultaneously, as all people experience constantly in any normal environment. A recent University of Wisconsin–Madison study found that the synergistic effects of pesticides and fertilizers at levels commonly found in groundwater can significantly impair the immune and endocrine systems as well as neurological health, with multiple consequences.[11] The researchers said the study adds to a growing body of evidence that current testing methods required for the registration and use of chemical pesticides are fundamentally flawed. The lead author of the study, Warren P. Porter, a UW–Madison professor of zoology and environmental toxicology, stated that "Neurological, immune and endocrine tests for pesticides have been mandated by federal law for almost three years, but there has been no enforcement of these laws."

Notes

1. McCampbell, Ann, M.D. *Multiple Chemical Sensitivity,* 1992, 1998. Available from Environmental Health Connection, 12 Bryce Court, Belmont, California 94002. $4 per copy. Checks payable to Ann McCampbell, M.D.

2. Ashford, Nicholas, and Claudia Miller. *Chemical Exposures: Low Levels and High Stakes, Second Edition,* New York: John Wiley & Sons, Inc., 1998.

3. *Ibid.*

4. Hu, Howard, M.D., M.P.H., ScD., Associate Professor, Harvard School of Public Health, "SPECT Scans and MCS," presentation at a University of Washington and Washington State Department of Labor and Industry conference, Chemicals, the Environment and Disease: A Research Perspective, May 7, 1999, Seattle, Washington.

5. Dager, S.R., J.P. Holland, D.S. Cowley, and D.L. Dunner. 1987. "Panic Disorder Precipitated By Exposure to Organic Solvents in the Work Place." *American Journal of Psychiatry,* 144, 1056–1058.

6. Finn, R. 1987–88. "A Review: Organic Solvent Sensitivity." *Clinical Ecology* 5, 155–158.

7. Morrow, L.A., et al. 1993. "Psychiatric Symptomatology in Persons with Organic Solvent Exposure." *Journal of Consulting and Clinical Psychology,* 61, 171–174.

8. Morrow, L.A., et al. "A Distinct Pattern of Personality Disturbance Following Exposure to Mixtures of Organic Solvents." *Journal of Occupational Medicine,* Vol. 31, No. 9, pp. 743–746, September 1989.

9. California State Department of Health Services, Behavioral Risk Factor Surveillance System (BRFSS) study of 4,000 randomly selected adults statewide, first in 1995 and replicated in 1996, in press with *American Journal of Epidemiology,* 1999.

10. New Mexico Department of Health, 1997 study of 1,814 randomly selected adults statewide.

11. Carlson, Ian H., James W. Jaeger, and Warren P. Porter, 1999. "Endocrine, Immune, and Behavioral Effects of Aldicarb (Carbamate), Atrazine (Triazine) and Nitrate (Fertilizer) Mixtures at Groundwater Concentrations." *Toxicology and Industrial Health,* Volume 15, No. 1–2, January–March 1999, p. 133–50.

Appendix C:
Starting Points for Finding Medical, Emotional and Social Support

Formal and informal MCS support networks exist across the country. The following resources are intended to be starting points that will lead you to additional resources and help you to locate MCS-aware physicians, support groups or individuals with MCS in your area who can offer local information and referrals. These are just a few of the many organizations and groups serving people with MCS. Most of them are run by volunteers who have the illness. It is recommended that you contact at least several groups for information. Each offers a different perspective. Comparisons can be helpful.

People at many of the organizations can refer you to MCS-knowledgeable individuals or organizations near you. Almost any contact you make will lead to more referrals if you ask: Do you know anyone who can refer me to a contact person in my area? Depending on where you live, you may locate support resources convenient to your location through your first contact, or you may have to follow up on several referrals before you are successful. Don't give up. A little detective work will usually pay off. If you get no answer or you reach someone who is having difficulty due to a chemical exposure, call another contact person. There are people willing to talk with you about coping with MCS either in person or by telephone or on the Internet.

Regional MCS newsletters are published in numerous states and

*cities. Some of the organizations listed below can tell you if there is
a regional publication in your area, or ask your local support group.
It is highly recommended that you also subscribe to at least one or
two of the national newsletters listed below.*

Information and Referrals

CHEMICAL INJURY INFORMATION NETWORK (CIIN)

This organization maintains an extensive list of MCS support
groups across the country, attorneys who represent clients in chemical injury cases, and a roster of physicians who recognize MCS and
physicians who can testify for MCS patients in court. Membership
includes subscription to *Our Toxic Times*, a monthly newsletter
with a focus primarily on medical, research and political issues associated with MCS and other toxic injuries. It is the most widely circulated MCS newsletter in the U.S. and advertises many products
and services for chemically sensitive people, housing ads, personal
requests for information and much more. The CIIN also maintains
a huge private library of resource materials on more than 1,000
MCS-related topics, primarily chemical, medical and legal issues.
By request they will send you a bibliography of resources on the topic
of your choice. Copies of the studies, articles or book chapters can
then be purchased from CIIN, or located through your local library
or other source.

> Editor: Cynthia Wilson
> P.O. Box 301
> White Sulphur Springs, MT 59645-0301
> Phone: 406-547-2255
> Web site: http://ciin.org
> Annual subscription fee: donation in any amount.

ENVIRONMENTAL HEALTH CENTER

An MCS treatment center that will provide physician referrals
in U.S., Canada and other countries. A health educator on staff will
answer questions by telephone or via the center's Web site. They
have published a book, *Less Toxic Alternatives*, as a resource guide
for all sorts of MCS-aware organizations and products; available for

$16 through the American Environmental Health Foundation (see below under "Mail Order Products for the Chemically Sensitive").

8345 Walnut Hill Lane Suite 220
Dallas, TX 75231
Phone: 214-368-4132
Web site: http://www.ehcd.com

MCS: HEALTH & ENVIRONMENT

Membership in this organization includes a subscription to *CanaryNews*, a quarterly newsletter that offers more resources than I can even begin to mention—all kinds of booklets, articles, and reprints, most of which are available to members for free or minimal fees and a self-addressed stamped envelope. Non-members pay $1 per request. Up to ten requests can be mailed in one return envelope. Members also receive an annual Resource Directory that also provides a wealth of MCS information: resources on EMF sensitivity; dentistry; legal aid; government agencies; resources for safe food and other products; useful books, documents and periodicals; Web sites; medical professionals; an index of audiotapes, videotapes and published material available to members through the lending library; a membership list and much more. Because this organization is based in Chicago, many of the resources listed are in Illinois, but the directory is still invaluable to anyone with an interest in MCS issues.

Membership $20; reduced fees and scholarships available by request.

Web site: www.mcshealthenviron.org

To join, make your check out to MCS: Health & Environment
Mail to: John Truskowski
251 Kimberly
Lake Forest, IL 60045

MCS INFORMATION EXCHANGE

By sending a self-addressed stamped envelope to this organization you will receive information for ordering a video tape, *Multiple Chemical Sensitivity: How Chemical Exposures May Be Affecting Your Health*, featuring interviews with people who have MCS and six doctors. You also will receive information on how to order the document *Statistical Results of a Survey of the Experience of 351 MCS Patients with 160 Therapies*.

Alison Johnson
2 Oakland St.
Brunswick, ME 04011

NATIONAL COALITION FOR THE CHEMICALLY INJURED (NCCI)

A coalition of support groups across the U.S.

2400 Virginia Ave. NW, Suite C-501
Washington, DC 20037

Contact people:

520-536-4625 Susan Molloy
301-897-9614 Lawrence Plumlee
847-776-7792 (Summer) Alice Osherman
941-756-1606 (Winter) Alice Osherman

HUMAN ECOLOGY ACTION LEAGUE, INC. (HEAL)

Has support group chapters located across the U.S. Publishes *The Human Ecologist*, a quarterly newsletter. Annual membership fee: $26.

P.O. Box 29629
Atlanta, GA 30359
Phone: 404-248-1898
E-mail: HEALNatnl@aol.com
Web site: http://members.aol.com/HEALNatnl/index.html

NATIONAL CENTER FOR ENVIRONMENTAL HEALTH STRATEGIES (NCEHS)

Referrals, policy development, research and advocacy. Expertise in indoor air issues, rights of those disabled by chemical/environmental exposures, public and commercial buildings access issues, accommodations in the workplace and more. Provides info package, media packages, educational materials and speakers bureau. Member of the President's Committee on Employment of People with

Disabilities. Publishes *The Delicate Balance*, a quarterly newsletter with a focus on indoor air quality, chemical sensitivities and related environmental and public health issues. Membership: $15 individual, $10 limited income, $20 family, $25 business/professional.

Mary Lamielle, President
1100 Rural Ave.
Voorhees, NJ 08043
Phone: 856-429-5358
E-mail: ncehs@ncehs.org

MCS Referral & Resources, Inc.

Focuses on recognition, prevention and research of multiple chemical sensitivities and carbon monoxide disorders. Provides professional outreach resources, patient support resources and information on MCS evaluation, accommodation, treatment and research. Copies of published literature available for library processing fee. Request selected bibliography.

Albert Donnay, President of Board of Directors
508 Westgate Rd.
Baltimore, MD 21229-2343
Phone: 410-362-6400
Fax: 410-362-6401
Web site: http://www.mcsrr.org

Ecological Health Organization and Action Coalition

Affiliate of the National Center for Environmental Health Strategies. Non-profit advocacy, support and referral organization for people who have MCS and others who care about preventing this illness. Bi-monthly newsletter. Fee: $15, includes Resource Directory; $7 low income; Resource Directory only $5.

Editor: Elaine Tomko
P.O. Box 0119
Hebron, CT 06248-1119
Phone: 860-228-2693

SHARE, CARE AND PRAYER

A nonprofit Christian organization encouraging, educating and equipping the environmentally sensitive and those with chronic fatigue syndrome, candidiasis and fibromyalgia. No set fee for newsletter and other materials. Donations help to cover expenses. Send a written request for a New Member Packet. You will receive Environmental Illness Basic Resource information, Bare Basics Diary for identifying triggers, order forms for cassette tapes, videotapes and other resources that are unique to this organization.

Executive Director: Janet Dauble
P.O. Box 2080
Frazier Park, CA 93225
Web site: http://www.sharecareprayer.org

Counseling

There are several avenues for finding MCS-aware counselors. You can get local referrals from doctors in your area who recognize MCS. The organizations listed above may also be able to make referrals. Some mental health professionals advertise their services in Our Toxic Times *and other newsletters, and may offer telephone appointments. You may also get personal referrals for good counselors who are not aware of MCS, but would be open to accommodating you and learning about MCS issues. To get a sense of which counselor you would like to work with, talk with several by telephone and ask any questions you may have about their qualifications, experience with clients who have MCS or other disabilities, and what type of therapy they practice (supportive, psychoanalysis, spiritual, family systems, behavioral). It also can be helpful to meet with more than one counselor in person before you make a decision regarding who to work with. Some counselors will meet with you for a few minutes at no charge to introduce themselves.*

Spiritual Support

Many churches and spiritually oriented groups provide spiritual direction or counseling to individuals by request. Many spiritual directors also work in private practice. Some are non-denominational, others are associated with specific religious or non-religious groups. The following are two Christian-based resources. For additional resources contact a church, synagogue or organizations in your area that promote the spiritual or religious orientation of your choice. Friends, support group members, health food stores and independent book stores are other potential sources of referrals.

SHARE, CARE AND PRAYER

See information above under "Information and Referrals"

HAND OF HOPE COUNSELING MINISTRY

Christian counseling. Office hours 11–5 Mountain Time.

Chaplain Jim Forbes and Jan Forbes, R.N.
RR 1
Box 135-B
Hot Springs, SD 57747
Phone: 605-673-5565

Online Support Groups

The Web sites for online MCS support groups, e-mail lists, newsgroups and chat rooms change from time to time. Those listed here were current at the time of publication. The best way to locate online support is to visit MCS-related Web sites that provide links. The Washington State MCS Network and the Environmental Health Network (see "Miscellaneous Resources" below) are two examples.

CHEMICAL-ILLNET NEWSGROUP

Chemical-Illnet newsgroup is an Internet community where the chemically ill, friends and family can get information and support and learn how to become proactively involved in advocating for accommodation and acceptance of MCS. Andi DesJardins, list owner, has a Web page at http://www.herc.org/. There is a link in the drop down menu to "Newsgroups." Subscription information also available by going to The Gathering Place at http://www.herc.

org/together/home.htm and click on "Newsgroups." Or contact chemxpose@aol.com or webmaster@herc.org by e-mail for information.

MCS-CI-EXILE

An international, unmoderated discussion forum for those with MCS who wish to move forward in understanding and coping with MCS. Issues addressed include: family and social; medical; research; health care; economic; workplace; educational; political; environmental; advocacy, legal; accommodations; lifestyle and government. To access: http://www.egroups.com/group/MCS-CI-exile or hhtp://home.wtal.de/nodi/MCS-CI-exile/.

Health Care Providers

Many different types of physicians and alternative practitioners can be helpful to patients with MCS. The best way to find out which ones recognize this illness is to ask other people with MCS in your area. Get a variety of recommendations, opinions and perspectives. Each physician or practitioner will have certain areas of expertise and will have different strengths and weaknesses. The following organizations can refer you to a doctor in your area who recognizes MCS.

AMERICAN ACADEMY OF ENVIRONMENTAL MEDICINE (AAEM)

Referrals to physicians who specialize in the treatment of environmental illness.

7701 E. Kellogg, Suite 625
Wichita, KS 67207
Phone: 316-684-5500
Web site: http://www.AAEM.com

CHEMICAL INJURY INFORMATION NETWORK (CIIN)

See information above under "Information and Referrals"

MCS: HEALTH & ENVIRONMENT RESOURCE DIRECTORY

See information above under "Information and Referrals"

ENVIRONMENTAL HEALTH CENTER, DALLAS

See information above under "Information and Referrals"

Electrical Sensitivity Information and Resources

The following organizations can provide additional resources and recommend books for further reading.

THE EMR ALLIANCE

410 West 53rd St. Suite 402
New York, NY 10019

SWEDISH ASSOCIATION FOR THE ELECTROSENSITIVE

Web site: http://www.feb.se/

Mail Order Products for the Chemically Sensitive

NATIONAL ECOLOGICAL AND ENVIRONMENTAL DELIVERY SYSTEM (NEEDS)

527 Charles Ave., Suite 12-A
Syracuse, NY 13209
Call for a catalog, toll free: 1-800-634-1380, or visit their Web site at http://www.needs4u.com.

AMERICAN ENVIRONMENTAL HEALTH FOUNDATION

8345 Walnut Hill Lane, Suite 225
Dallas, TX 75231
Call for a catalog; toll free number for orders: 1-800-428-2343; or 214-361-9515 for information.

Miscellaneous Resources Referred to in the Narratives

WASHINGTON STATE MCS NETWORK

Washington State MCS Network provides a wealth of information on resources in Washington state and far beyond. Provides links to online support groups with subscribers all over the globe.
Web site: http://members.aol.com/WSMCSN/
E-mail: WSMCSN@aol.com

ENVIRONMENTAL HEALTH NETWORK (EHN)

Publishes *The New Reactor* newsletter
Editor: Barbara Wilkie
P.O. Box 1155
Larkspur, CA 94977-1155
Support and Information Line: 415-541-5075
Web site: http://users.lanminds.com/~wilworks/ehnindex.htm

NATIONAL AMERICAN INDIAN ENVIRONMENTAL ILLNESS FOUNDATION

135 NE Barron Dr. #B-203
Oak Harbor, WA 98277
E-mail: tchansen@gte.net

SAFE SCHOOLS

Irene Wilkenfeld is an environmental health consultant, lecturer and writer specializing in issues related to the sick school syndrome. Her consulting company provides in-service training workshops for school districts, educating them about the myriad health hazards in schools and offering efficacious and cost-effective options to detoxify schools. Wilkenfeld also offers phone consultations and personalized research reports to help students, parents and teachers advocate for change and win accommodations. Wilkenfeld is passionate that every school must be a citadel of safety.

Irene Wilkenfeld
Web site: http://www.head-gear.com/SafeSchools/

ECOLOGICAL HEALTH ALLIANCE

This registered charitable self-help organization provides a variety of resources, information and support groups. Membership includes subscription to their quarterly newsletter, *Ecological Health Alliance Support News*. Fee: $25; reduced fee for those in need. Make check payable to AEHA-BC Branch.

Allergy and Environmental Health Association–B.C. Branch
Box 30033 Saanich Centre PO
Victoria, BC V8X 5E1
Message phone: 250-658-2027

HEALTHY HOUSING COALITION OF NEW MEXICO

Provides information about New Mexico, upcoming events, MCS information, safe housing tips and more. They do not provide housing.

P.O. Box 53184
Albuquerque, NM 87153
Phone: 505-989-2565
Web site: http://www.herc.org/hhc/
E-mail: hhcmail@aol.com

Appendix D:
Recommended Reading

Many books are available on MCS and related topics. Here are a few that offer good overviews and bibliographies for further information.

Allergic to the Twentieth Century: The Explosion in Environmental Allergies—From Sick Buildings to Multiple Chemical Sensitivity. Peter Radetsky. Boston: Little, Brown, 1997. Provides an overview of the sufferers, skeptics and scientists engaged in the movement toward awareness of MCS and Gulf War illness.

An Alternative Approach to Allergies: The New Field of Clinical Ecology Unravels the Environmental Causes of Mental and Physical Ills. Theron G. Randolph and Ralph W. Moss. New York: HarperCollins, 1990. Written by the first modern physician to diagnose and treat environmental illness.

Chemical Exposures: Low Levels and High Stakes, Second Edition. Nicholas A. Ashford and Claudia S. Miller. New York: John Wiley & Sons, Inc., 1998. Reviews the medical data on MCS. Addresses causes of MCS, health effects associated with chemicals and foods, possible physiological mechanisms, diagnostic approaches, recent developments in research and recognition, an Environmental Exposure and Sensitivity Inventory. Written by an MIT professor, and a physician and assistant professor at the University of Texas.

Chemical Sensitivity: A Guide to Coping with Hypersensitivity Syndrome, Sick Building Syndrome and Other Environmental Illnesses. Bonnye L. Matthews. Jefferson, NC: McFarland, 1992.

Chemical Injury and the Courts: A Litigation Guide for Clients and Their Attorneys. Linda Price King. Jefferson, NC: McFarland, 1999. The guide addresses in detail several important areas of chemical injury and the legal process: defining problems and solutions; examining available resources; cultivating a knowledge of chemical-related diseases and injuries; and facilitating effective attorney-clent relationships and case strategies. Leading attorneys contribute case studies and essays offering perspectives on chemical injury and the law.

Defining Multiple Chemical Sensitivity. Edited by Bonnye L. Matthews. Jefferson, NC: McFarland, 1998. Contains chapters written by a psychologist, an attorney and two physicians with expertise in MCS. A medical section addresses porphyria, SPECT scan studies, and psychological issues related to MCS. A legal section discusses how one state's workers' compensation system fails workers in a toxic age. A personal section discusses the author's experience in the workers' compensation system; science and the literature is addressed in yet another section.

Environmentally Induced Illnesses: Ethics, Risk Assessment and Human Rights. Thomas Kerns, Jefferson, NC: McFarland, [in press]. Addresses the ethics of managing environmental health and ubiquitous toxicants (such as solvents, pesticides and artificial fragrances). The work includes recent medical literature on chronic health effects from exposure to toxicants and the social costs of these disorders; relevant historic and human rights documents; recommendations for public policy and legislation; and primary obstacles faced by public health advocates.

Is This Your Child? Discovering and Treating Unrecognized Allergies in Children and Adults. Doris J. Rapp, M.D. New York: William Morrow, 1991.
Is This Your Child's World? How You Can Fix the Schools and Homes That Are Making Your Child Sick. Doris J. Rapp, M.D. New York: Bantam Books, 1996. These two books are written by a renowned medical expert on children and allergies and environmental illness.

Multiple Chemical Sensitivity. Ann McCampbell, M.D. Self-published, 1998. A booklet providing simple answers in laymen's terms to some commonly asked questions about MCS: What is MCS? Who gets it? What causes it? What are the symptoms? How is it diagnosed? How is it treated? What is the political history of the illness? Available by mail order only: Environmental Health Connection, 12 Bryce Court, Belmont, CA 94002. $4 per copy. Discount available when ordering ten or more copies. Make checks payable to Ann McCampbell, M.D.

Multiple Chemical Sensitivity: A Survival Guide. Pamela Reed Gibson. Oakland, CA: New Harbinger Publications, 1999. Features survival tools for coping with many aspects of MCS: coping with the life impact of a chronic illness and with the unique aspects of MCS; the need for social support, medical intervention and environmental controls; self-help options; identity and psychological issues; applying for disability benefits and much more.

Sauna Detoxification Therapy: A Guide for the Chemically Sensitive. Marilyn G. McVicker. Jefferson, NC: McFarland, 1997. Sauna detoxification therapy for MCS patients is covered, including case studies of MCS sufferers who have chosen sauna treatment. The unique requirements for a home sauna whose construction materials are suitable for MCS patients, and how to build one, are presented. Includes a directory of organizations and vendors.

Staying Well in a Toxic World: Understanding Environmental Illness, Multiple Chemical Sensitivities, Chemical Injuries and Sick Building Syndrome. Lynn Lawson. Self-published, 1993. Crammed with resources, references, suggested readings and information. Almost an encyclopedia of MCS issues and where to find more information on every topic featured—laboratories that test for toxic chemicals in the human body, dozens of resources for safe products, who to turn to if you work in a sick building, actions to protect yourself from fragrance exposures, tips for protecting your children from toxics, A Bill of Rights for the Chemically Injured ... the list goes on and on. $15.95 plus $3 shipping/handling. Make check payable to Lynn Lawson and mail to: Staying Well, P.O. Box 1732, Evanston, IL 60201.

Taking Charge, How to Master the Eight Most Common Fears of Long-Term Illness. Irene Pollin, M.S.W., with Susan K. Golant. New York: Times Books, 1994. An excellent book on coping with any long-term illness. Offers practical tools for addressing family issues related to the illness, mastering the fear of loss of control and self-image, fear of dependency, fear of stigma, fear of abandonment and more.

Tired or Toxic? A Blueprint for Health. Sherry Rogers, M.D. Syracuse, NY: Prestige Publishing, 1990.

Index